Clinical Text Mining

Hercules Dalianis

Clinical Text Mining

Secondary Use of Electronic Patient Records

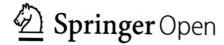

Hercules Dalianis
DSV-Stockholm University
Kista, Sweden

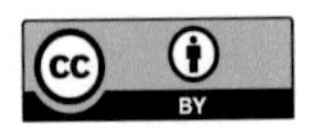

ISBN 978-3-030-08715-9 ISBN 978-3-319-78503-5 (eBook)
https://doi.org/10.1007/978-3-319-78503-5

Softcover re-print of the Hardcover 1st edition 2018

Printed on acid-free paper

This Springer imprint is published by the registered company Springer International Publishing AG part of Springer Nature.
The registered company address is: Gewerbestrasse 11, 6330 Cham, Switzerland

In Memory of Kostas Pantazos
Στη μνήμη του Κώστα Παντάζου

Preface

Objectives

Patient records are written by the physician during the treatment of the patient for mnemonic reasons and internal use within the clinical unit, but the patient record is also written for legal reasons.

Today a very large number of patient records are produced in the healthcare system. The patient records are mostly in electronic form and are written by health personnel. They describe initial symptoms, diagnosis, treatment and outcomes of the treatment, but they may also contain nursing narratives or daily notes.

In addition, patient records contain valuable structured information such as laboratory results, blood tests and drugs. These records are seldom reused, most likely because of ignorance, but also due to a lack of tools to process them adequately, and last but not least, there are ethical policies that make the records difficult to use for research and for developing tools for physicians and researchers. There is a plethora of reasons to unlock and reuse the content of electronic patient records, since they contain valuable information about a vast number of patients who have been treated by highly skilled physicians and taken care of by well-trained and experienced nurses. Over time a massive amount of patient record data is accumulated where old knowledge can be confirmed and new knowledge can be obtained.

This book was written since there was a lack of a textbook describing the area of clinical text mining. The healthcare domain area is complex and can be difficult to apprehend. There are plenty of specialised disciplines in healthcare. Applying text mining and natural language processing to health records needs special care and understanding of the domain. This book will help the reader to quickly and easily understand the health care domain. Some issues that are treated in this book are: What are the problems in clinical text mining and what are their solutions? Which are the coding and classification systems in the health care domain? What do they actually contain and how are they used? How do physicians reason to make a diagnosis? What is their typical jargon when writing in the patient record? Does jargon differ between different medical specialities?

This book will give the reader the background knowledge on the research front on clinical text mining and health informatics, and specifically in healthcare analytics. It is valuable for a researcher or a student who needs to learn the clinical research area in a fast and efficient way. A book is also a valuable resource for targeting a new natural language in the domain. Each additional language will add a piece to the whole equation.

The experiences described in this book originate mainly from research that utilised over two million Swedish hospital records from the Karolinska University Hospital during the years 2007–2014. The general aim was to build basic tools for clinical text mining for Swedish patient records and to address specific issues. These tools were used to automatically:

- detect and predict healthcare associated infections;
- find adverse (drug) events; and
- detect early symptoms of cancer.

To accomplish this, the text in the patient records was manually annotated by physicians and then different machine learning tools were trained on these annotated texts to simulate the physicians' skills, knowledge and intelligence. The book is also based on the extensive source of scientific literature from the large research community in clinical text mining that has been compiled and explained in this book.

This book will also describe how to get access to patient records, the ethical problems involved and how to de-identify the patient records automatically before using the records, and finally, methods to build tools that will improve healthcare.

The research question of this 10-year research project are many fold, and started with the general research question(s):

- Using artificial intelligence to analyse patient records: Is it possible and will it improve healthcare?

This actually can be distilled to several research questions of which one is of special interest:

- Can one process clinical text written in Swedish with natural language processing tools developed for standard Swedish such as news paper and web texts to extract named entities such as symptoms, diagnosis, drugs and body parts from clinical text?

This major issue can then be subdivided into the following questions:

- Can one decide the factuality of a diagnosis found in a clinical text? What does *Pneumonia?* or *Angina pectoris cannot be excluded* or just *No signs of pneumonia?* really mean?
- Can one determine of the temporal order of clinical events? Have the symptoms occurred a week ago or two years ago?

- Can new adverse drug effects be found by extracting relations between drug intake and adverse drug effect?
- How much clinical text must be annotated manually to obtain correct and useful results?
- How can patient privacy be maintained while carrying out research in clinical text mining?

Organisation of Book Chapters

This book contains 12 chapters, of which Chaps. 1–4 are more general, Chaps. 5–8 are technical, Chap. 9 contains ethical issues and finally Chap. 10 describes various applications. More specifically Chap. 1 gives a short introduction of the research area clinical text mining. Chapter 2 continues with the history of the patient records and the languages used in them. Chapter 3 is about the use of patient records and the requirements the different health professionals, such as physicians and nurses, have on the patient record system. The electronic patient record system is also described. Chapters 2 and 3 are easy to read for anyone who is interested in the area and do not require any technical or medical background knowledge. Chapter 4 specifically describes the linguistic characteristics of patient record text in the form of spelling errors, domain specific abbreviations, negation and assertion expressions, etc. for English, Swedish and other languages.

Chapter 5 presents the different medical classifications and terminologies as ICD diagnosis codes, SNOMED CT, MeSH, UMLS, ATC etc. Chapter 6 describes the metrics for the evaluation of information retrieval and natural language processing systems, the annotation techniques and evaluation metrics and the concepts of training, development and evaluations sets for information retrieval systems. Chapter 7 presents the basic building blocks for clinical text processing, which are almost identical to the building blocks for standard text processing using natural languages processing techniques but adapted for medical text. The content of this chapter is similar to the content in a textbook on computational linguistics but much more condensed.

Chapter 8 presents the computational methods for text analysis and text classification, including both rule-based and machine learning-based methods such as unsupervised and supervised methods. Unsupervised methods include distributional semantics and clustering. Supervised methods such as *Support Vector Machine, (SVM)* and *Random Forest* are presented. This chapter also describes the knowledge representation of text in various formats suitable for computational methods. Active learning is described that is used for selecting appropriate training material for the machine learning algorithms. The chapter continues with a presentation of ready and half ready toolboxes to use. Chapter 9 discusses ethics and other ethical issues while working with sensitive material, such as patient records, and how to apply for ethical permission and the safe storage of sensitive data. The chapter continues with a description of automatic de-identification (sometimes called anonymisation) of patient record text as well as pseudonymisation of patient records, the risk of re-identification of de-identified patient records when adding more databases to the data set and how to avoid re-identification by using so-called privacy preserving linkage.

Chapter 10 presents various applications of clinical text mining. Applications include those for patients and laypersons as well as those for clinicians working with patients, clinical researchers and administrators within hospital management, at both the county council level and national level. All these applications utilise the electronic patient record text as input data.

Chapter 11 describes the different fora and conferences for clinical text mining and finally Chap. 12 summarises the lessons learned from the previous chapters and also makes some concluding remarks.

Intended Readers

The intended readers of this book are researchers, PhD-students and students at an advanced level in computer science and health informatics. The intended reader may also be a person who will start working in the area of clinical text mining and needs to obtain access to clinical data and initiate research in the domain, but also personnel in commercial business who will start building applications in clinical text mining.

Limitations

The book has a computer science orientation specialising in computational linguistics and data science applied on electronic patient records. It does not deal with healthcare but with methods, tools and applications for assisting healthcare personnel. The book does not treat requirement engineering nor business models in computer science, nor speech recognition of speech in the clinical domain.

Book Project During Sabbatical Stay in Sydney

The initial parts of this book commenced in January 2016 when applying for funding for a sabbatical stay at Commonwealh Scientific and Industrial Research Organisation (CSIRO) and Macquarie University in Sydney, Australia. Dr. Cecile Paris and Dr. Diego Molla had previously jointly invited the author to CSIRO and Macquarie University. The aim was to have a quiet and stimulating place to work in while writing this book.

Most parts of this book were written during the sabbatical stay in Australia in the Australian spring of 2016, the winter of 2016–2017 and the autumn of 2017 (in the southern hemisphere the seasons are the opposite of the seasons of northern hemisphere).

The following research institutes were visited during the sabbatical stay in Australia: CSIRO/Macquarie University in Sydney, CSIRO at the Australian eHealth Research Centre (AeHRC) in Brisbane, the Centre for Health Informatics, Australian Institute of Health Innovation (AIHI) at Macquarie University in Sydney, the Capital Markets Cooperative Research Centre (CMCRC) in Sydney and the Australian National University in Canberra, and the company HLA Global in Sydney. The research in this book was presented and chapters in the book were discussed, missing parts of the book were filled in.

In addition to the research work carried out on Swedish electronic patient records: the Stockholm Electronic Patient Record (EPR) Corpus contained in the HEALTH BANK—Swedish Health Record Research Bank, an extensive literature study was carried out. Of course today it is difficult to cover and find everything: moreover only literature published in English, or translated to English, and literature written in Swedish was included.

Aims

The intention of this book is to be a source of knowledge for mining of clinical text, describing applications of data science using as input clinical texts including pathology reports and providing an understanding of ethical and security issues when working with clinical data.

The importance of this book is that there are large repositories of electronic records which are never reused and at the same time there is a large demand for tools that can make healthcare better and more efficient. Examples of these tools are detection and prediction of healthcare associated infections, and drug related adverse side effects, but also detection of early symptoms of cancer using the large number of patient records.

Acknowledgements

First I would like to thank all the members of my research group the Clinical Text mining group at the Department of Computer and Systems Sciences (DSV) at Stockholm University in Kista, Sweden. In the order of appearance: Martin Duneld, Sumithra Velupillai, Gunnar Nilsson, Mia Kvist, Maria Skeppstedt, Aron Henriksson, Claudia Ehrentraut, Hideyuki Tanushi, Alyaa Alfalahi and Rebecka Weegar, but also other collegues in my close surrounds, such as Henrik Boström, Panos Papapetrou, Lars Asker, Jussi Karlgren, Fredrik Olsson, Aurélie Névéol,

Alicia Pérez, Jon Patrick, Anthony Nguyen, Bevan Koopman, Sarvnaz Karim, Frédérique Segond, Hélène Metzger, Viggo Kann, Joakim Nivre, Arne Jönsson, Joakim Dillner, Karin Sundström, Jan Nygård, Øystein Nytrø, Dimitris Kokkinakis, Søren Brunak, Ingvar Krakau and many others. Specific thanks to Maria Skeppstedt, Sumithra Velupillai, Aron Henriksson, Rebecka Weegar, Hanna Suominen and Tina Dalianis who gave very valuable comments on early versions of this book and to Olympia Tsaknaki for her comments on the English. I also would like to thank the very competent anonymous copy editor from Springer who read through the final manuscript and gave valuable comments on the language.

Thanks to Cecile Paris and Diego Molla for inviting me to CSIRO and Macquarie University in Sydney and for their team's warm and friendly atmosphere.

Thanks to Erik Thuning in the Datamaskinscentralen (DMC) at DSV and the hardworking people there for their support with the servers. Thanks also to Elda Sparrelid, Gunnar Ekeving and Bo Vikström at Karolinska University Hospital in Stockholm for helping with the permissions for accessing patient records, extracting data and arranging confidential agreements.

Thanks also to my wife Kerstin for joining me to Australia. I was not sure you wanted to come with me to Sydney but I did not need to persuade you! Thanks also to our lovely two daughters, Freja and Hera, who also came along to Australia on different occasions!

Riksbankens Jubileumsfond is acknowledged for funding this project.

Sydney, Australia
Athens, Greece
Sigtuna, Sweden
January 2018

Hercules Dalianis

Contents

Chapter 1
Introduction

The amount of digitised data available from healthcare systems is increasing exponentially. This data is seldom reused, either due to ignorance of its potential importance or due to the lack of available tools to process the data, but also because of the ethical policies regarding access to sensitive data. Healthcare systems and specifically health record systems contain both structured and unstructured information as text. More specifically, it is estimated that over 40% of the data in healthcare record systems contains text, so-called clinical text, sometimes also called electronic patient record text (Dalianis et al. 2009).

Clinical text contains valuable information about symptoms, diagnoses, treatments, drug use and adverse (drug) events for the patient that can be utilised to improve healthcare for other patients. The physician also writes her or his reasoning for the conclusion of the diagnosis of the patient in the patient record (Groopman 2007).

However, clinical text also contains sensitive information such as personal names, telephone numbers and addresses of the patient and relatives. This information needs to be pseudonymised before the clinical text can be utilised for secondary use (Velupillai et al. 2009).

A large amount of the information in an electronic patient record system is unstructured in the form of free text.

Clinical text is written by various professionals such as physicians, nurses, physiotherapists, psychologists etc. Often it is written under time pressure, and contain misspellings, non-standard abbreviations and jargon, as well as incomplete sentences, and is therefore difficult to process for natural language processing (NLP) tools developed for ordinary text, such as news text or text produced for a large number of readers (Allvin et al. 2011; Smith et al. 2014). Plenty of research has been carried out for clinical text processing for text written in English, but not that much for small and under resourced languages such as for example Swedish (Névéol et al. 2018). Nevertheless, a number of projects have been carried out at DSV, Stockholm University, during the years 2007–2017 in the area of clinical text mining in Swedish.

H. Dalianis, *Clinical Text Mining*, https://doi.org/10.1007/978-3-319-78503-5_1

Karolinska University Hospital has contributed over two million patient records from the years 2007–2014 to the Clinical Text Mining Group at DSV. This patient database, called HEALTH BANK—Swedish Health Record Research Bank, has obtained seven different ethical permissions for seven research projects that have been carried out or are ongoing. An initial publication by Dalianis (2014) described these efforts, and the experience from these efforts. This publication has been developed, extended and synthesised to this textbook.

This book will however, first go back in time, explaining the historical origin of the patient record, both papyrus and paper based, and the structure and content of the patient record. It will then continue with the first computer based patient record systems and examples of experimental patient record systems. The need and requirements for electronic patient record systems from clinical personnel including physicians and nurses will be described.

The process of obtaining access to electronic patient records for research will be explained, and will include applying for ethical permission, as well as practical issues regarding extracting, storing and using the patient records for research.

Natural language processing (NLP) will be explained and how information retrieval and text mining relates to NLP. Various tools for processing the patient records will be presented and the challenges in constructing these tools discussed. Challenges creating useful manually annotated data for training for so-called supervised learning will be described, in contrast to using various resources that are not annotated beforehand to train the system or artefact, so-called unsupervised learning. More specifically supervised learning simulates the behaviour of the human annotator for an artefact or system. The *annotator* is a person that manually will mark up data for training a machine learning system. *Active learning* will be used to select the most optimal data for annotation. System and artefact will be used interchangeably in this book. Algorithm is also used, but in this context as part of a system or artefact. Sometimes also the concept tool or application will be used.

The same annotated data can partly be set aside for evaluation of the artefact. There are various evaluation methods that can be used, for example k-fold cross validation, but also methods to calculate the significance of the results. These techniques are important for calculating the behaviour of the system and will be explained in this book.

First of all, to make electronic patient record text available for research, or for developing and testing applications, the records need to be de-identified since they contain information that can identify individual patients. One important application that will be described in this book is therefore the de-identification of electronic patient record text to de-identify the sensitive information, which means to remove information such as patient names, addresses and telephone numbers in the text that would otherwise reveal the identity of the patient. The identified sensitive information can be replaced with surrogates or pseudonyms, so that the text looks realistic without having any strange gaps and hence making the text coherent.

Once this first task is completed, then one can continue with the task of trying to address specific issues and attempt to acquire more knowledge.

Detecting adverse drug events (ADEs) is an example of a specific application area. An ADE may occur when a patient is treated for a disorder and can result from the use of one or more drugs and lead to the patient developing another disorder or symptom caused by the drug or drugs.

Predicting healthcare associated infections is yet another example of a specific application area that will be described in this book. A HAI is an infection that may occur while treating the patient at a hospital. It usually occurs when the patient is admitted to the hospital or just after being discharged, but according to its definition, the patient must have been admitted for at least 48 h (Ducel et al. 2002).

Other examples of specific applications that will be described are tools that may detect early symptoms of cancer, before the cancer has been detected or diagnosed. Some symptoms are very vague, but by having access to a large set of previous cancer cases with a lot of patterns, future cases may potentially be detected and predicted.

All these applications are based on analysing both the structured data of the patient record as well as the unstructured text using natural language engineering technology, or what also sometimes is called Artificial Intelligence.

Another, type of application is the handling of specific data. For example a pathology report is written by pathologists that have examined tissues from the human body to determine the disease the patient is suffering from. The result of the examination is written in free text in a pathology report that is given to the treating physician so he or she can decide on the treatment of the patient. For statistical reasons and for research the contents of the pathology reports are also entered into cancer registries, this is usually carried out manually by well-trained coders and is very time consuming work. The process of entering the content of the pathology report into a cancer registry can be automatised and in this book some examples will be provided.

Automatic diagnosis code assignment for discharge letters is another application that will be discussed: a secondary use of the same developed tool is for use for the validation of already assigned diagnosis codes. Diagnosis codes are assigned for the medical personnel as well as for administrative purposes, to calculate the cost of treatment and for the future planning of the overall healthcare provided by the whole clinical unit or hospital.

Automatic structuring of the patient record so it becomes more readable is another interesting application that will be explained. Automatic structuring will be carried out by either extracting the most important information and presenting it in a marked up format in the form of a hypertext, or by summarising the patient record.

Moreover, there is also the possibility to simplify the patient record so that a layperson can also understand it. This is because in some countries the patients have access to the patient record on the Internet and can read it, but the record is difficult to understand. However, there are ways to simplify the contents of the clinical text and explain expressions so a layperson can also understand the patient record.

In summary, we can conclude that there are many challenges in the area of clinical text mining, as well as important basic techniques that need to be explained.

Useful methods and their potential applications will be described and demonstrated, and finally summarised in this book in clinical text mining.

1.1 Early Work and Review Articles

One of the first articles written regarding clinical text mining is the article by Pratt and Pacak (1969), where the authors outline what is needed for the automatic processing of a clinical text in English to obtain an interpretation of the content.

More recently, two excellent reviews of clinical text mining are: Meystre et al. (2008), describing the state of the art of the research area, and Meystre et al. (2010), presenting the status of tools for de-identifying patient records. Yet another review article describing the detection of adverse drug events using text and data mining techniques is by Karimi et al. (2015b), while Freeman et al. (2013) review a number of tools for detecting healthcare associated infections and Spasić et al. (2014) compare different tools for detecting cancer symptoms. Regarding the closely related area biomedical text mining, see the textbook by Cohen and Demner-Fushman (2014).

The contents of this book will have as a starting point the work described by Dalianis (2014) but will extend with research work carried out by the author during 2014–2016 as well as work carried out by other contemporary researchers. This book also treats ethical and security issues, and details regarding various clinical text mining tools. Electronic patient records are written in different languages. Languages included in this book are Swedish, English and several European languages, as well as Japanese and Chinese.

Other important articles that describe the state of the art in the research field are: Nguyen et al. (2010), Skeppstedt et al. (2014) and Velupillai et al. (2014).

Regarding SNOMED CT, there are two articles describing the use of the terminology, (Lee et al. 2013, 2014), but the articles focus on academic publications and not so much on practical implementations using SNOMED CT.

Chapter 2
The History of the Patient Record and the Paper Record

This chapter introduces the long history of the patient record, from ancient times until now. From the Egyptians in 1600 BC to the Greeks with Hippocrates, *the father of medicine*, to the Arabs and then to the Age of Enlightenment in Europe and the development of natural sciences during the eighteenth century. From the first attempts to describe and classify nature that formed the first patient record, to the modern paper based records with their distinct headlines and sections describing the findings and symptoms, treatment of the patient and finally the outcome; followed by the organisation of the paper records to make them easy to follow. This chapter will also discuss the Greek-Latin terminology in the patient records.

2.1 The Egyptians and the Greeks

The first known record is Egyptian from 1600 BC, but it is not a proper patient record, rather a written document on papyrus describing surgical treatment of war wounds. The document lists a number of cases and is probably part of a textbook (Al-Awqati 2006). The document is also called the Edwin Smith Papyrus, see Fig. 2.1.

Then followed the Greeks with Hippocrates, sometimes called *the father of medicine*, who was active 2400 years ago at the god Asclepius' temple of healing on the island of Kos in today's eastern Greece. Hippocrates considered medicine as a science separated from religion and magic. Hippocrates took careful notes of his patients about symptoms, appearance of the patient, social situation etc. to decide on the treatment, he also recommended that these documents should be stored and used by new physicians involved in the treatment of the patient (Cheng 2001).

Hippocrates also introduced the oath, in Greek *Όρκος* or Hippocratic Oath, that all physicians should use and follow. The oath is still used today by physicians (North 2002; Winau 1994). The Hippocratic Oath also contain principle of confidential information given by the patient to the physician, which should be kept by

H. Dalianis, *Clinical Text Mining*, https://doi.org/10.1007/978-3-319-78503-5_2

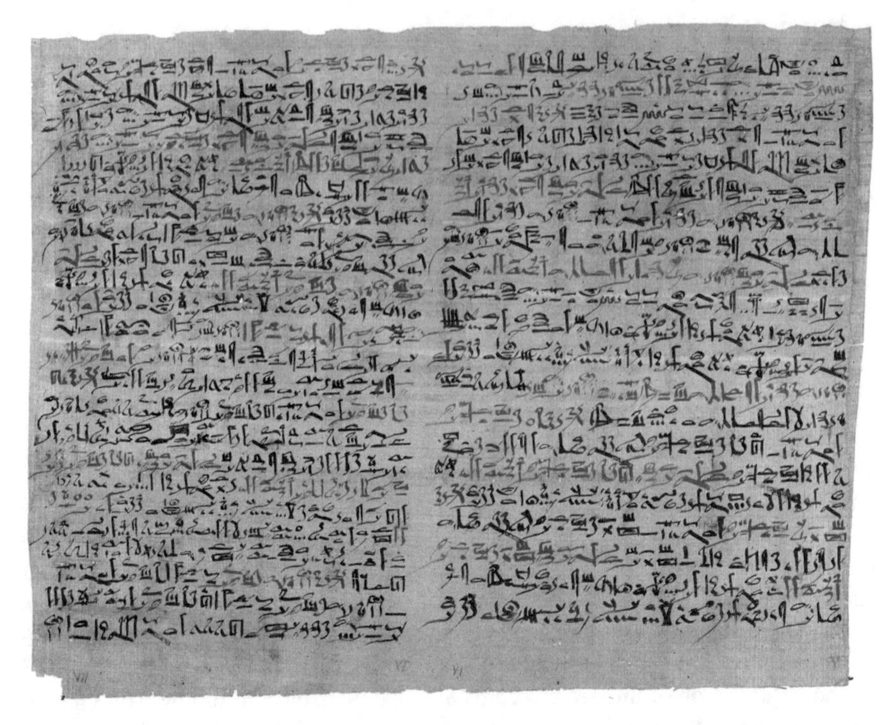

Fig. 2.1 Part of the Edwin Smith Papyrus describing in Egyptian hieratic script (a cursive hieroglyph writing) different surgery cases from 1600 BC (Published in Wikipedia)

the physician and not revealed to anyone else not involved in the treatment of the patient. Moreover, one more important guiding principle is that the physician should not harm the patient while treating him or her.

There are over 42 case histories that originate from Hippocrates, and were written down several hundred years after Hippocrates' death. These case histories describe symptoms day by day for a typical patient and the outcomes, most of them leading to the death of the patient.

Aelius Galenus, Claudius Galenus or just *Galen of Pergamon* should also be mentioned since he was a famous Greek physician, medical writer and philosopher living from 129 AD to 199 AD during the Roman Empire. Galen wrote extensive literature of the diseases and treatment of patients. Galen's writing influenced and dominated medicine in the Western world until the fourteenth century, i.e. for over 1300 years!

The Byzantine Empire from c. 330 AD to 1453 AD was the bridge between the Greco-Roman medicine and Arab or Islamic medicine. Specifically the Byzantine Greek physician Paul of Aegina, or Paulus Aegineta, who lived in 700 AD wrote the medical encyclopedia Medical Compendium in Seven Books, which later was translated to Arabic from Greek. This work was used for 800 years and was printed in Venice 1528 (Temkin 1962).

2.2 The Arabs

The knowledge of Greek medicine was kept and developed by the Arabs into so-called *Islamic Medicine* during the Islamic Golden Age, from the eighth century to the thirteenth century. The Arabs introduced the concept of hospital and the use of hospitals. They also were the first to keep written records of patients and their medical treatment. Students were responsible for keeping the patient records, which were later edited by doctors and referenced in future treatment (Miller 2006; Syed 2002).

2.3 The Swedes

With the evolution of natural science in early eighteenth century during the Age of Enlightenment in Europe, everything in nature was classified and described. The most famous representative of this was the Swedish scientist, botanist and physician Carl Linnaeus, (in Swedish Carl von Linné), who built up a whole classification system for naming organisms. Linné is also known as the *Father of modern taxonomy* and was active in the early eighteenth century at Uppsala University in Sweden.[1]

In the same environment and time period the Swedish physician Nils Rosén von Rosenstein was active, he applied for the position of lecturer, *adjunct*, at the faculty of Medicine at Uppsala University but to obtain this position the condition was that he must travel to study in Europe and also obtain a doctoral degree in medicine which was not possible in Sweden at that time. 1728 Rosén von Rosenstein obtained a scholarship to undertake his studies, as well as absence of leave from his teaching assistant position, with a full salary to travel in Europe. During 3 years he visited leading German, French, Swiss, Italian and Dutch universities including the famous Leiden University in Holland. He stayed in Geneva for 9 months and obtained medical training. In 1730 he defended his doctoral thesis in medicine with the title *De historiis morborum rite consignandis*, in English translated to *The correct documentation of the disease progression*, at the University of Harderwijk in Holland. The dissertation treated the principles of medical record writing and included the whole patient and his or her surroundings. Apart of Rosén von Rosenstein's impressions from his study trip in Europe he was probably inspired that scientists at that time, including Carl von Linné, were diligently classifying nature in written form.

Finally to become a lecturer in Medicine at Uppsala University he was required to make a dissertation test and he carried it out by writing a small thesis with the title *De usu methodi mechanicae in medicina*, in English *The use of mechanical methods in medicine*.

[1]Carl Linnaeus, https://en.wikipedia.org/wiki/Carl_Linnaeus. Accessed 2018-01-11.

In 1740 Nils Rosén von Rosenstein became a professor of medicine at Uppsala University and started the first formal education in medicine in Sweden. Rosén von Rosenstein refurbished the *Nosocomium academicum*, later the Uppsala Academic Hospital. The hospital was very small, probably with only eight beds. Rosén von Rosenstein introduced the taking of careful notes of his patients, their symptoms, diagnosis and treatment as well as their social condition. The patients were mostly poor people.

The first formal medical record system in Sweden was developed and systematic medical documentation was introduced in connection with the opening of the Serafimerlasarettet (Seraphim Hospital) in Stockholm in 1752, (Nilsson and Nilsson 2003; Nilsson 2007)

In Sweden the paper based patient record system was developed and refined until 1980 when computerised patient record systems started to become more common and it was more or less completely digitalised by 2007, (Nilsson 2007). See Chap. 3.3 for more details about the early electronic patient record systems in Sweden.

For a description of the historical development of the patient record see also Gillum (2013).

2.4 The Paper Based Patient Record

Patient records are written for several reasons, for the physician as a memory support, but also to be used by other physicians involved in the healthcare process of the patient. Clinicians such as nurses, physiotherapists, dieticians, psychologists etc. are also involved in writing in the patient record. Since the nurses usually take care of the patient on a daily basis they also write daily notes in the patient record, while the physicians make notes at certain time points. The other reason for documenting the healthcare process of a patient is for legal reasons, since it is required by law in many countries.

Patient records have many different names, for example patient record, health record, case sheet, and case history. A paper based record contains certain distinguishable parts: the identity of the patient, the reason for the visit, the history and background of the patient (*anamnesis*, the results of *physical examination, current symptoms* (status), *assessment* and *treatment*, time points of documentation, the result of the treatment, the *discharge letter* (Greek επίκρισις decision, judgement, in Swedish *epikris*) and who has written the record, see Fig. 2.2 (Nygren and Henriksson 1992; Nilsson 2007).

During the doctor's visit the physician listens first to the anamnesis from the patient, the physician then checks for symptoms, trying to exclude possible symptoms, leading to a *diagnosis*, containing the name of the disease and the possible *body part* where the disease is situated. Symptom is interchangeble with *finding* in this book, as well as disease is used interchangeably with *disorder*.

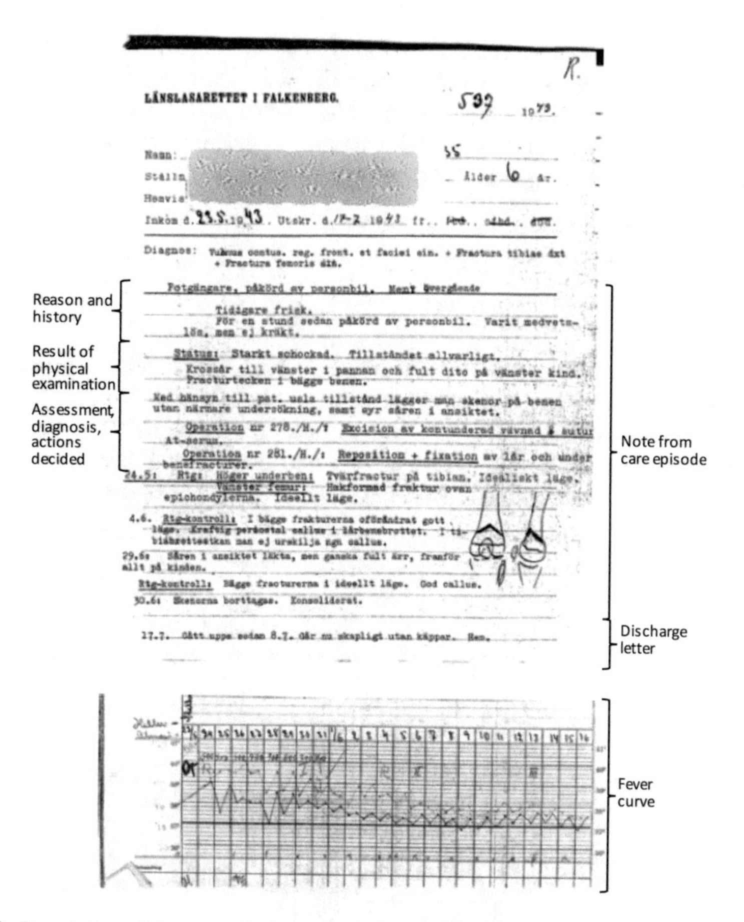

LÄNSLASARETTET I FALKENBERG.

Namn:
Ställn.
Hemvis
Inkom d. 23.5.1943. Utskr. d. 1943 fr.

Ålder 6 år.

Diagnos: Vulnus contus. reg. front. et faciei sin. + Fractura tibiae dxt + Fractura femoris sin.

Fotgängare, påkörd av personbil.

Tidigare frisk.
För en stund sedan påkörd av personbil. Varit medvetslös, men ej kräkt.

Status: Starkt schockad. Tillståndet allvarligt.
Krossår till vänster i pannan och fult dito på vänster kind.
Fracturtecken i bägge benen.

Med hänsyn till pat. usla tillstånd lägger man skenor på benen utan närmare undersökning, samt syr såren i ansiktet.

Operation nr 278./M./ Excision av kontunderad vävnad & sutur
At-serum.

Operation nr 281./M./: Reposition + fixation av lår och underbensfracturer.

24.5: Rtg: Höger underben: Tvärfractur på tibian. Idealiskt läge.
Vänster femur: Hakformad fraktur ovan epichondylerna. Ideellt läge.

4.6. Rtg-kontroll: I bägge frakturerna oförändrat gott läge. Kraftig periostal callus i lårbensbrottet. I tibiabrottetskan man ej urskilja ngn callus.

29.6: Såren i ansiktet läkta, men ganska fult ärr, framför allt på kinden.

Rtg-kontroll: Bägge fracturerna i ideellt läge. God callus.

30.6: Skenorna borttages. Konsoliderat.

17.7. Gått uppe sedan 8.7. Går nu skapligt utan käppar. Hem.

Fig. 2.2 Description of the parts of a Swedish medical record from 1943. A 6 year old boy was hit by a car and obtained a fracture on his femur. He was treated for this for 6 weeks on the hospital, and then discharged from the hospital when he could walk again. (The whole health care episode fits into a one page.) (© Läkartidningen, 2010-04-12, number 15 (http://www.lakartidningen.se/OldWebArticlePdf/1/14161/1003.pdf. Accessed 2018-01-11.) All rights reserved—reprinted with permission from Läkartidningen)

For patients admitted to the hospital the patient record contains daily notes of the status and progress of the treatment. These notes are usually taken by the nurses who also take daily care of the patient.

The discharge letter should contain a summary of the whole healthcare period, with instructions on how the patient should be taken care of after discharge from the hospital.

There are several ways to write a medical record: one is the source oriented patient record that it is divided based on the source of the information; one is the physician', the nurse', the laboratory or the radiology results and various other sources.

Another well-known model is the *Problem Oriented Medical Record (POMR)*, (Weed 1968). The model is based on an early decision on the main problem or problems of the patient, thereafter each problem is assessed on a daily basis without loosing focus on the patient. The SOAP model originates from the POMR model (Cameron and Turtle-Song 2002). *SOAP* stands for:

- *Subjective* (anamnesis, actual reasons for visit).
- *Objective* (findings when observing).
- *Assessment* (analysis).
- *Plan* (treatment and healthcare plan).

The paper record file gets thicker the more visits the patient has made. One observation is that older paper record sheets may have a different color e.g. more towards yellow than newer records, which shows how long time the patient may have been visiting the hospital for. The paper record file may also have red time stamps and the distance between them indicates the level of problems a patient may have, see Fig. 2.3.

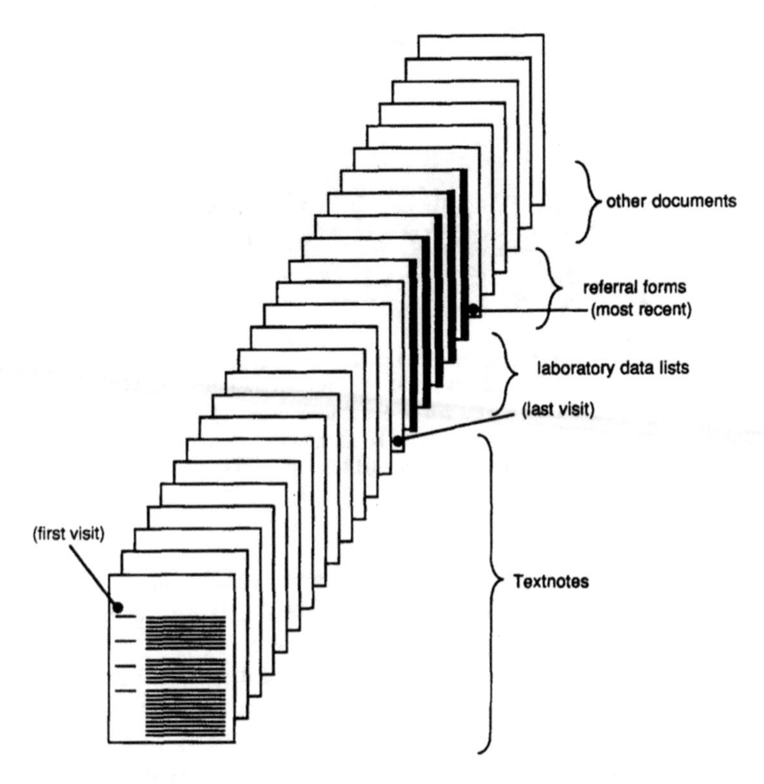

Fig. 2.3 The different parts of the medical record in a timeline, there can be another order of the paper record where the last visit is in the beginning of the file (© 1992 Elsevier Inc. All rights reserved—reprinted with permission from Elsevier Inc. Published in Nygren and Henriksson (1992))

Obviously it is difficult to analyse paper based patient records using computational linguistic methods, since the paper record needs to be scanned and the characters recognized with optical character recognition (OCR) techniques; however, in the next chapter we will demonstrate how to analyse electronic (digital) patient records.

2.5 Greek and Latin Used in the Patient Record

Greek language was obviously used by the Greeks in the early versions of the patient record and Greek physicians were famous during the antique period, both during Greek and later Roman rule. Many of the Greek documents were translated to Arabic by the Arabs after the fall of the western Roman Empire. The Arabs improved medicine a lot stretching over 500 years, during the Islamic Golden Age stretching from 700 to 1200 AD, and many of their manuscripts regarding medicine were translated to Latin. Many of the Arabic terms describing drugs and chemistry remained in their original form but Latinised.

Latin became the language of the scholars in the western world from 1000 AD. In the thesis by Nilsson (2007), she gives many examples of Swedish patient records using Swedish language to describe the status of the patient.

Generally pathological terms such as diseases and symptoms are written with Greek vocabulary, and anatomical terms such as body parts where the disease occurs are written with Latin vocabulary.

In Swedish many of these foreign terms are adapted to Swedish morphology using Swedish inflections, the so-called *swedification* for medical terms in Swedish, the same for English, German and French (Grigonytė et al. 2016).

Regarding swedification of medical terms in Swedish, by Grigonytė et al. (2016), write that prefixes are less affected by swedification than suffixes which are more common and therefore adapted to Swedish morphology. An example is the Greek-Latin medical term *cholecystitis* "gallbladder inflammation" that is written *koleocystit* in Swedish. Using the Swedish *k* in the prefix instead of *c* and removing the *-is* in the suffix.

In an article by McMorrow (1998) there is an interesting overview of the road of Greek-Latin medical terminology through the Islamic Golden Age and the medieval Europe into the nineteenth century.

2.6 Summary of the History of the Patient Record and the Paper Record

This chapter discussed the origin of patient records from ancient times to now, the reasons for producing patient records, the structure of patient records, the different distinct parts, how the records were filed and stored, and the POMR and SOAP models used to structure the patient record, but also the language they are written in and the influences and use of Greek and Latin. The different languages they are written in influence each other in orthography and inflections of terms. This is important to know for the understanding of how the electronic patient record systems of today are structured and work.

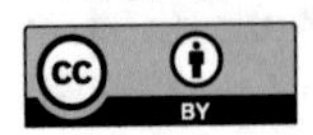

Friedman and Hripcsak (1999) continue to elaborate on future systems and future directions where NLP will be used to assist physicians. Examples that are given include the automatic assignment of ICD-9 codes to patient records. Continuous voice recognition will assist the physician in entering text to the patient records, simultaneously the patient record will be encoded in the standard codes using standard terminology.

A important review article by Meystre et al. (2008) makes a nice overview of many systems available (in 2008), and possible directions that these systems will be developed in.

In a study by Velupillai and Kvist (2012), the authors present three scenarios consisting of *adverse event surveillance, decision support alerts* and *automatic summaries* where clinical text mining is used.

Finally, in an article by Jensen et al. (2012) the authors elaborate on disease trajectories and predictions based on big data mining of electronic patient records.

3.3 Electronic Patient Record System

The official bibliographical term is *electronic patient record (EPR)*, other names are electronic health record (EHR), electronic medical record (EMR), computerised patient record, digitised patient record or just health record. Another name is case sheet. The electronic patient record does not live by itself but in a computerised system, which is called electronic patient record system (Åhlfeldt et al. 2006).

The first electronic patient record systems in Sweden were constructed in the mid 1960s and 1970s as a series of pilot tests at Karolinska University Hospital, specifically at the Thorax clinic (chest clinic). These early electronic patient record systems had no real impact on the healthcare.

The first system used was called Costar and came from the high-tech, advanced, academic environment of Harvard University, Massachussets, USA: the system was developed and was later called Swedestar in Sweden and Finnstar in Finland.

Later in the 1980s a lot of systems were developed both inhouse at the primary care level and later at hospitals, and also involving local companies. In parallel with this was the development of first automation of the chemistry laboratories, which also was a driving force to use an electronic patient record system. These systems were also well received by the clinicians since they were involved in giving feedback, while later when the large centralised system arrived the clinicians did not feel that they really were involved in the requirements engineering process (Kajbjer et al. 2010). Kajbjer et al. (2010) have a nice overview of the different systems and the growth of the electronic patient record systems in Sweden from 1988 to 1995, and how the large variety of suppliers finally was refined down to four major suppliers.

One early study describes the requirements engineering process for the Karolinska Hospital Information System, it shows the basic information that should be included in such a medical record system and how the data should be stored in a database so it can be updated and retrieved easily (Mellner et al. 1974).

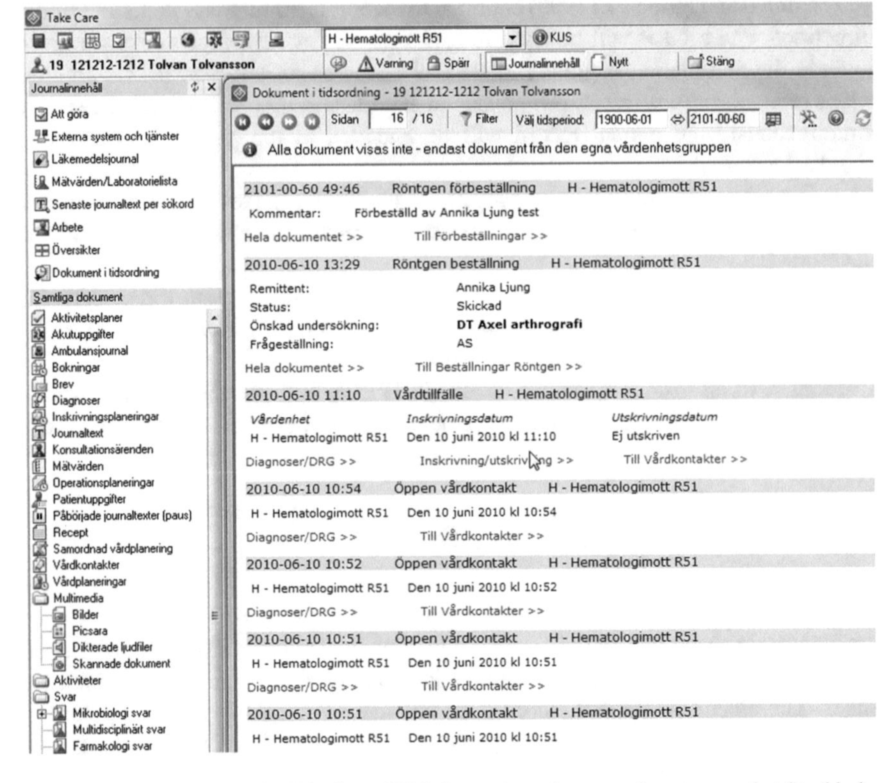

Fig. 3.1 Screenshot from the TakeCare CGM electronic patient record system used at Stockholm County Council (Stockholms läns landsting, SLL)

The paper based patient record has become digitised, in electronic health records systems, without in some cases, really improving the ways the physician can browse in it, see Fig. 3.1.

The improvements are mainly that the record is available faster when digitised than obtaining it in paper form from the archive, where the paper record file had to be fetched by the assistant and sometimes the file was missing in the archive. In the electronic patient record the laboratory results, X-ray images etc. are also directly available and other physicians located at other places involved in the healthcare process of the patient can easily access the patient record. A radiology report is written by the radiologist and is an interpretation in text of the X-ray image.

In Metzger et al. (2012) there is an interesting overview of the number of electronic patient record systems in use in contrast to paper based system, where the USA and Canada are at the bottom in the western world with only 46 and 37% respectively, together with France (where 68% of French general practitioners use EHRs) while Norway and New Zealand with 97% use of electronic patient records systems; of course now in 2017 these numbers must have changed.

Many of the previous ways of observing the paper file have disappeared in the electronic patient record system. However, there has been research in how to improve the ways to browse the patient record. Early work included LifeLines (Plaisant et al. 1998), where the patient record is presented in a timeline where the physician can browse back in time and can easily observe what findings (problems), diagnosis and drugs (medications) have been documented; the physician can also click (or zoomin) on the medications and obtain more details on the type of medications, see Fig. 3.2.

In an interesting article by Roque et al. (2010), the authors compare six different prototype electronic patient record systems that propose different viewing systems for temporal data. The systems studied are LifeLines, Lifelines2 (the extension of LifeLine), Timeline, CLEF KNAVE-II and finally AsbruView. Lifelines2 and CLEF can also be used by clinical researchers. CLEF has built-in automatic generation of summaries. The conclusion is the systems need to improve the way the granularity of the data is presented. Since much of the data stored in patient record systems is in textual form, different text mining tools would be appreciated for presenting the semantic content of the patient records. We can consider Lifelines2 and CLEF as the new type of electronic patient record that can search the whole patient record repository to perform *cohort studies*. Cohorts are groups of individuals with similar characteristics, such as disease, drug use, age, gender etc.

3.4 Different User Groups

The current and possible user groups of advanced electronic patient record systems are firstly, of course, clinicians such as physicians, nurses, physiotherapists, dieticians and psychologists treating individual patients. Secondly clinical researchers, medical researchers, pharmacologists and epidemiologists studying cohorts of patients (that is groups of patients with similar characteristics, social parameters, geographical information or location), but also data scientists for development of new tools. Thirdly hospital management and administration, along with national health board officials. lastly the business world, such as pharmaceutical companies and electronic patient records system suppliers for development of systems.

3.5 Summary

This chapter summarised the user needs and presented the different user groups in medical healthcare such as clinicians, clinical researchers, hospital management and administration, the business world and data scientists. The needs of clinicians accessing, reading and writing the patient record, previously in paper form but now in electronic form were described along with the first attempts to use natural language processing of the patient record. The chapter also described the difference

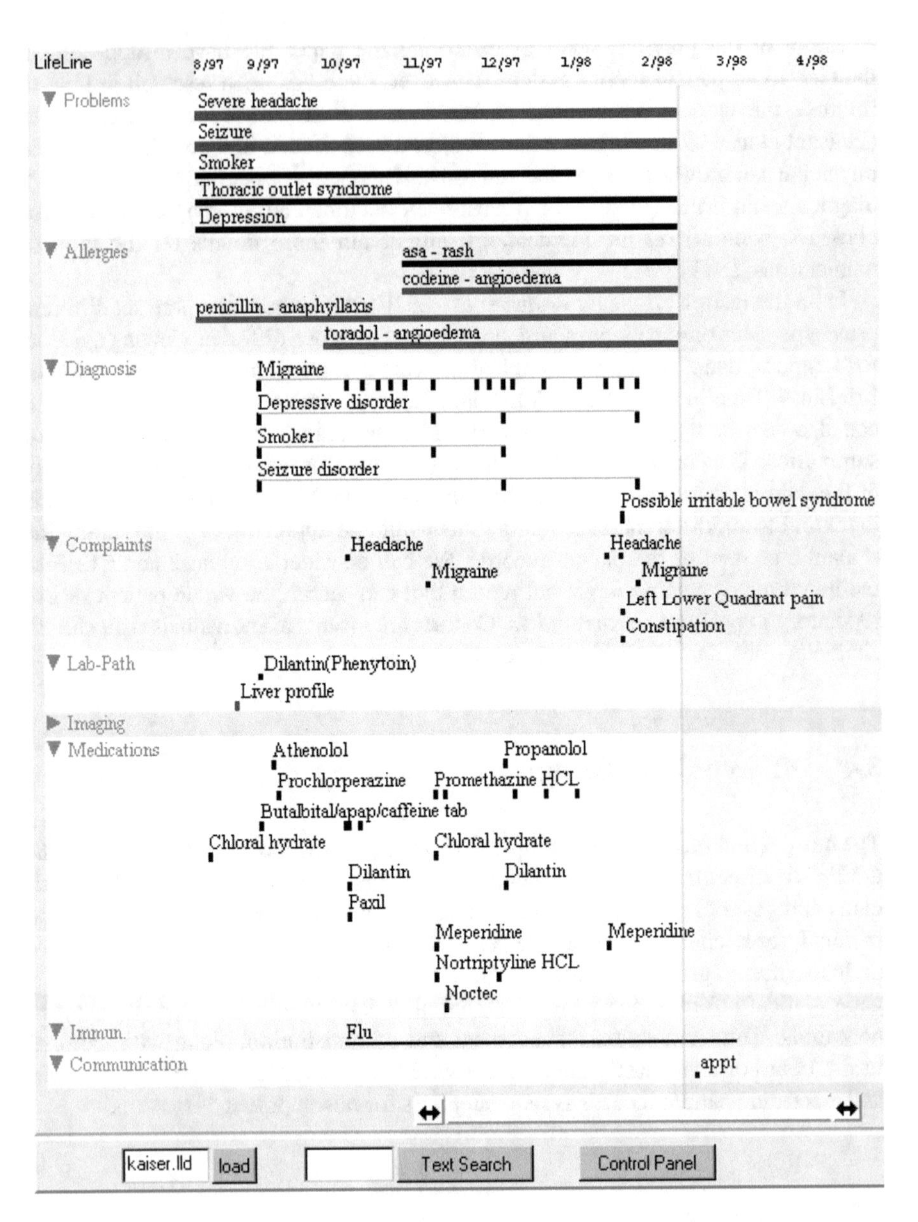

Fig. 3.2 Screenshot of the Lifelines (Lifelines, http://www.cs.umd.edu/hcil/lifelines/kaiserlifelines.jpg. Accessed 2018-01-11.) prototype electronic patient record system

between individual patient record access (LifeLines prototype) and accessing all patient records (Lifelines2 prototype) in the repository, and the reason for studying several patient records simultaneously to predict the future and collect statistics. The need to present various prototypes for clinicians to show them the possibilities of medical healthcare information systems was also discussed.

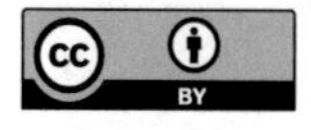

Chapter 4
Characteristics of Patient Records and Clinical Corpora

This chapter will describe the characteristics of patient records compared to other text types including: A comparison of the characteristics of patient records written in different languages, the number of spelling errors compared to other types of text, syntactic differences, word choices, abbreviations, acronyms, compounds and compound construction, negation expression and also speculative cues and factuality expressions in clinical text. Patient record text is different from standard text such as news text or novel text regarding style and grammatical correctness. Patient record text is also written by many different professionals with different writing skills. The varies writing style depending on whether it is a physician's note or a discharge letter, or nursing narratives. Also the style varies between different clinical units and specialities. Pathology reports in turn contain a very special type of writing, where the physician describes a sample taken from the patient without ever meeting the patient.

4.1 Patient Records

Patient records are primarily written for hospital internal use and for mnemonic reasons. Daily running notes might contain more spelling errors or noisiness than discharge letters that are read by a larger audience (Ehrentraut et al. 2012).

The linguistic term *corpus* meaning a document collection, the plural *corpora* means several document collections.

In a study comparing Finnish and Swedish nursing narratives the authors observed a large number of linguistic and grammatical errors in both languages. Complete sentences are rare; auxiliary verbs such as *be, is* and *are* are rarely used. *Patient* is not mentioned unless in abbreviated form, or sometimes the patient as a subject is not mentioned at all, the subject of the sentence is also missing, a sentence may contain only a number of adverbs such as *fever, sweating, trouble breathing* (Allvin et al. 2011).

H. Dalianis, *Clinical Text Mining*, https://doi.org/10.1007/978-3-319-78503-5_4

Septisk pat, oklart fokus, rundodlas före Zinacef.
(in Eng. Septic pat, unclear origin, roundcultured before Zinacef)

which means:

Patienten har sepsis med oklart ursprung, bakterieodling tas från samtliga möjliga infektionsfokus, inklusive blododling, innan behandling med Zinacef inleds.
(in Eng. The patient has sepsis of unclear origin, bacterial culture samples taken from all possible foci for infection, including blood culture samples, before commencing treatment with Zinacef.)

Fig. 4.1 An example of aggregated clinical text. It has been rephrased so as not to contain any redundant information, and it presumes background knowledge of the reader (© 2014 Springer International Publishing Switzerland—reprinted with permission. Published in Dalianis (2014))

According to Pakhomov et al. (2005) there are 30% non-word tokens, abbreviations, acronyms, misspellings, wrongly used grammar etc. in clinical text, which is a good indication of the noisiness of clinical text.

Generally patient records are written by highly skilled physicians and nurses using domain specific terms. For example, patient record text is very domain specific depending on which medical discipline it is written in. Each discipline or domain within medicine uses its own set of terms that can be incomprehensible by other disciplines.

Patient records are, as mentioned in Sect. 2.4, highly structured with headings such as *Subjective, Objective, Assessment* and *Plan*, but this is not always followed by individual physicians, or between different professions. The writing under the correct heading and also the names of the headings may differ in different clinical units or hospitals. The same for different electronic patient record systems.

The patient records are written under time pressure; the patient record systems do not contain any spelling correction (or grammar checking) system due to the difficulties of building such a function because of the complicated non-standard vocabulary used within healthcare.

Therefore, in clinical text non-standard abbreviations, domain specific acronyms, and incomplete sentences without a subject can be observed, meaning the patient is not mentioned, only his or her status. The text is short and efficient, and written in telegraphic style, see Fig. 4.1 on aggregated clinical text. Moreover, the text can be full of jargon and misspellings. The physicians reason and argue to find the diagnosis by excluding symptoms and mention them in negated form (Groopman 2007).

4.2 Pathology Reports

Pathology reports are written by pathologists, highly skilled physicians. Pathologists are experts in interpreting laboratory tests. They study samples and tissues from the human body, and describe the samples in free text in pathology reports. The structure and content of a pathology report is as follows: the name of the patient, how each tissue sample was obtained, how it looks compared to normal tissue and normal cells, the diagnosis and a description of the diagnostic tests such as (possible) tumor such as size (typically in mm or cm), type and grade in the *TNM scale* (growing and spreading risk of the tumor), lymph node status, number of lymph nodes containing tumor metastasis, the position in body (Asamura et al. 2014). Whether the tumor is non-invasive or invasive and contains various hormone receptors (for example Her-2), proliferation rate (Ki-67, MIB1) or Gleason grade (also called Gleason score) depending on cancer type and finally the tumor margins (when performing a biopsy the tumor size is not known).[1,2]

Generally, pathology reports are more carefully written than patient records, often with correct spelling. The pathology reports have more semi-structure than the patient records. The pathologist is using the writing and the text as a tool for their profession, see Fig. 4.2 for an example of a pathology report for breast cancer.

The pathology report is sent to the physician who is treating the patient, so the physician can decide how to proceed with the treatment.

Samples are taken from the body at regular intervals to follow the progress, or hopefully the regression, of the cancer. The pathology reports are very often registered in regional or national cancer registries for statistics on cancer treatment and outcomes.

At the cancer registry well-trained coders read and interpret the content of the pathology report and then manually enter the information to the cancer registry. This work is time consuming and tiresome. The agreement between pathology report coder is not known. One hypothesis is that agreement between them may be around 0.8 in F-score as for other annotation tasks.

4.3 Spelling Errors in Clinical Text

The number of spelling errors in clinical text has been calculated in a few publications. Ruch et al. (2003) found around 10% spelling errors in French clinical text, while Patrick and Nguyen (2011) only found 2.3% spelling errors in Australian English clinical text, and finally Nizamuddin and Dalianis (2014) found 7.6% spelling errors in the Stockholm EPR PHI Corpus containing in total 174,000 tokens. In another smaller subset of the same Swedish clinical corpora 1.1% of the words were found to be misspelled (Grigonyte et al. 2014).

[1] Contents of a pathology report, http://ww5.komen.org/BreastCancer/ContentsofaPathologyReport.html. Accessed 2018-01-11.

[2] National Cancer Institute, Pathology Reports, http://www.cancer.gov/about-cancer/diagnosis-staging/diagnosis/pathology-reports-fact-sheet#. Accessed 2018-01-11.

```
Mammaresektat (ve. side) med infiltrerende duktalt
karsinom, histologisk grad 3
Tumordiameter 15 mm
Lavgradig DCIS med utstrekning 4 mm i kranial
retning fra tumor
Frie reseksjonsrender for infiltrerende tumor (3 mm
kranialt)
Lavgradig DCIS under 2 mm fra kraniale
reseksjonsrand

ER: ca 65 % av cellene positive
PGR: negativ
Ki-67: Hot-spot 23% positive celler. Cold spot 8%.
Gjennomsnitt 15%
HER-2: negativ
Tidl. BU 13:

3 sentinelle lymfeknuter uten pÃěviste patologiske
forandringer
```

Translated to English:

```
Mamma specimen (le. side) with infiltrating ductal
carcinoma, histological grade 3
Tumor diameter 15 mm
Low-grade DCIS extending 4 mm in cranial direction
from the tumor
Free resection margins for infiltrating tumor (3 mm
cranially)
Low-grade DCIS less than 2 mm from the cranial
resection margin

ER: ca 65 % of the cells are positive
PGR: negative
Ki-67: Hot-spot 23% positive cells. Cold spot 8%.
Average 15%
HER-2: negative
Prev. BU 13:

3 sentinel lymph nodes without proven pathological
changes
```

Fig. 4.2 Extract from the free text part of an anonymised breast cancer pathology report in Norwegian (and its translation to English). The data in the figure is made up and can not be linked to any individual (© 2015, Association for Computational Linguistics (ACL). All rights reserved. Reprinted with the permission of ACL and the authors. Published in Weegar and Dalianis (2015))

In Fig. 4.3, shows a clinical text with a number of misspellings.

In Table 4.1 there are some examples of misspellings in Swedish patient record text and their correct spelling, together with the corresponding misspelled version in English and the correctly spelled English word.

Beklagar nissförstånd rek ayt provar mindre smaker som innehåller mindre Kolhydrater 8vilket pat benämner som smaken sött som diasip, komplett näring naturell samt provide x-tra tomat. Ut tar upp dessa till avd för utprovning . Vi ska se vad vi kna göra med de näringsdrycker som finns i hemmet då pat är åter hemma...

(in Eng; Sorry for the nisunderstanding rec tto try less flavours that contain less Carbohydrates 8which pat name as taste sweet like diasip, complete nutrition natural as well as provide x-tra tomato. Ut takes these to clin for try out . Let's see what we cna do with the nutrition drinks in the house when pat is back home. . .).

Fig. 4.3 Example of clinical text with spelling errors (© 2009 The authors—reprinted with permission from the authors. Published in Dalianis et al. (2009))

Table 4.1 Some examples on misspelled Swedish words in a patient record and their equivalents in English

Misspelled word Swedish	Correct word	Misspelled word Eng	Correct word Eng
K<u>ar</u>nvatten	Kranvatten	T<u>pa</u> water	Tap water
Deli<u>g</u>ation	Delegering	Deli<u>g</u>ation	Delegation
Reko<u>m</u>endation	Rekommendation	Reco<u>m</u>endation	Recommendation
Inge<u>r</u> förtroende	Inge<u>t</u> förtroende	Gives confidence	No confidence

Misspelled parts are underlined. The last *confidence*-example is a real example where the misspelling *inger* (gives) is a real word while the author wanted to write *ingen* (no), which is not obvious since it created a real word and changed the whole meaning of the expression

Table 4.2 Spelling errors in various types of text

Type of texts	Misspellings
Text written in e.g. Word	0.2
Newspaper text	0.05–0.44
Web text	0.8
Hand written text	1.5–2.5
Typed textual conversations	5.0–6.0
Patient record text	10.0

© 2012 The authors—reprinted with permission from the authors. Published in Ehrentraut et al. (2012)

In Table 4.2, taken from Ehrentraut et al. (2012), the percentage of spelling errors in patient record text compared with other type of texts can be observed. One finding by Ehrentraut et al. (2012) was that patient records contained twice as many abbreviations as text messages, with 10.6% and 5.0% respectively.

4.4 Abbreviations

An abbreviation is a way to write a word not using the complete spelling, for example the word *patient* written as *pat*. Abbreviations are an efficient way to write text, but it makes the reading slower since the reader has to interpret the abbreviations. In some cases the abbreviation can be ambiguous, for example, *pat* can be ambiguous since it also can mean *pathological.*

Here follow some studies on abbreviations in Swedish clinical text: in a study by Allvin et al. (2011), the authors found that 4.7% of the words in Swedish nursing narratives, a subset of the Stockholm EPR Corpus (Dalianis et al. 2009), were abbreviations. In a study by Isenius (2012), Isenius et al. (2012), 19,408 tokens from another subset of the Stockholm EPR Corpus were extracted and then manually annotated by a senior physician with previous experience in annotating clinical texts. In total 2050 tokens were identified as abbreviated tokens, of these 335 were unique. In total in this small subset 1% abbreviations were found. Skeppstedt et al. (2012) constructed a rule-based system to detect findings and disorders in a subset of the Stockholm EPR Corpus, 14% of the manually annotated disorders in the gold standard were written in an abbreviated format. Nizamuddin and Dalianis (2014) studied the Stockholm EPR PHI Corpus, which is a subset of the Stockholm EPR Corpus, and found 2.7% abbreviations. Finally, Olsson (2011) analysed patient records from a Swedish surgery department, and the author found 2.4% abbreviations.

Patrick and Nguyen (2011) found 0.7% abbreviations in Australian English clinical text. Wu et al. (2011) found in a small English clinical corpora containing 18,225 tokens a total of 1386 abbreviations, which is around 0.8% abbreviations.

Siklósi et al. (2014) studied a Hungarian clinical sub-corpus within ophthalmology consisting of 552,594 tokens and found 113,091 abbreviated tokens, which correspond to 20% of the total corpus.

Regarding ambiguity of the clinical abbreviations there are two studies: Liu et al. (2001) found that 33% of the abbreviations in English clinical text were highly ambiguous and Lövestam et al. (2014) analysed 40 different abbreviations in Swedish dietetics notes from the subset of the Stockholm EPR Corpus, written by three professions: dieticians, nurses and physicians. A contextual analysis showed that 33% of the abbreviations were ambiguous.

Many of the abbreviations, around 12%, in clinical text are compounds where one part is composed of an abbreviation and the other part of a complete word, see Table 4.3 for examples (Kvist and Velupillai 2014). For a dictionary of Swedish medical abbreviations see Cederblom (2005).

Table 4.3 Examples of Swedish clinical abbreviations from a Stockholm EPR Corpus, some of the them are ambiguous

Abbreviated word in Swedish	Resolved word in Swedish	Resolved word in English
ul	Ultraljud/underläkare	Ultrasound/assistant physician
rtg	Röntgen	X-ray
p5	Petrokantär femurfraktur	Hip fracture
Lungrtg	Lungröntgen	Lung X-ray

One abbreviation *lungrtg* (lung X-ray) is composed of a full word form *lung* and an abbreviation *rtg* meaning *röntgen* (X-ray)

Both the *Unified Medical Language Systems (UMLS)* and *Systematized Nomenclature of Medicine Clinical Terms (SNOMED CT)* contain abbreviations, and can be used for creating abbreviations lists. UMLS is only available for English, while SNOMED CT is available in several languages, but not all language versions contain abbreviations.

Many clinical words in Swedish are compounds, either full word form or combinations of full word forms and abbreviations as in the example *lungrtg* (lung X-ray).

4.5 Acronyms

Acronyms are a specialised form of abbreviations, usually using the first letters of each word in a phrase, or some combination of letters from words in a phrase forming an acronym with capital letters that also are easy to pronounce, while abbreviations consists of letters from one or more specific words, which are also easy pronounce.

An example of how an acronym has many different meanings is shown in Pakhomov et al. (2005). The UMLS concept *RA* has over 20 meanings, all of them different from each other, for example: *rheumatoid arthritis, renal artery, right atrium, right atrial, refractory anemia, radioactive, right aram, rheumatic arthriti, ragweed antigen, refractory ascites, renin activity, rheumatoid arthritis, renal artery, right atrium, right atrial, refractory anemia, radioactive, right aram* and *rheumatic arthritis*.

Patrick and Nguyen (2011) found 1.5% acronyms in Australian English clinical text. Kvist and Velupillai (2014) analysed both emergency unit records and radiology reports written in Swedish and found that 11% and 7.1% respectively contained abbreviations, and 33% and 55% respectively of the abbreviations where acronyms.

4.6 Assertions

Assertions are prepositions that have some sort of positive or negative polarity. They can range from completely negated to a speculative form through to a complete affirmed preposition.

4.6.1 Negations

Negations are very common in clinical text, since physicians use negations to exclude symptoms while reasoning about the cause of a patient's disease. The physician will write down the reasoning chain leading to the concluded disease; therefore, a lot of negated symptoms will be found in a patient record.

In a study by Chapman et al. (2001) more than half of the expressions in American radiology reports were found to contain negations. One explanation for this high amount is that these reports are mainly physicians' notes containing the physicians' reasoning (Groopman 2007). Physicians' notes contain more negations than nursing narratives that are about the daily healthcare of the patient. Another example is the English BioScope clinical corpus containing 13.6% negations (Vincze et al. 2008).

In Swedish, see Sect. 4.7.2 the texts from various clinical units under the heading *assessment* were studied and it was found that negated sentences or expressions encompassed 13.5% of the texts (910 negated sentences of a total of 6640 sentences) (Dalianis and Skeppstedt 2010).

4.6.2 Speculation and Factuality

Many of the expressions in clinical text are either negated or *uncertain* (sometimes also called *speculative*), or just asserted or assertions. Uncertain or speculative expressions in clinical text indicate that a statement is not affirmed or factual, and the uncertainty or level of speculation may range from slightly uncertain to strongly uncertain, see Fig. 4.4 for an example.

The English BioScope clinical corpus containing 6383 sentences was manually annotated for negation, speculation and scope. 13.4% of the sentences contained speculative keywords, so-called hedge sentences, and 13.6% contained negations, some of them overlapping (sentences containing both speculations and negations) (Vincze et al. 2008).

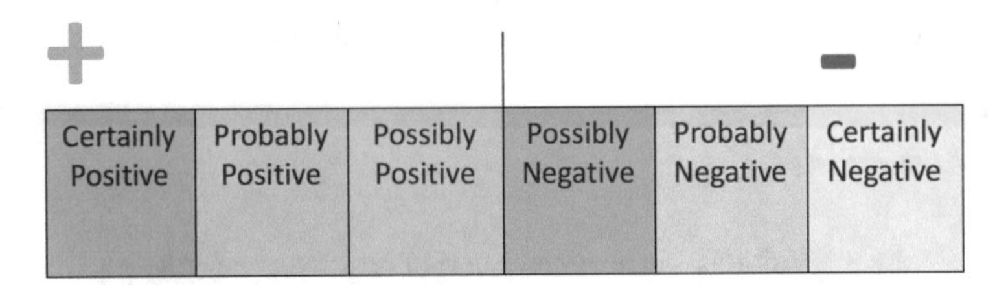
+
-
Certainly Positive
Probably Positive
Possibly Positive
Possibly Negative
Probably Negative
Certainly Negative
Patient has Parkinsons disease.
Physical examination strongly suggests Parkinson.
Patient possibly has Parkinson.
Parkinson cannot yet be ruled out.
No support for Parkinson.
Parkinsson can be excluded.

Fig. 4.4 Examples of different levels of certainty, ranging from completely affirmed to negated (© 2012 The author—reprinted with permission from the Author. Published in Velupillai (2012) p. 34)

A Swedish clinical corpus called the Stockholm EPR Diagnosis Factuality Corpus was developed to study uncertainty levels related to diagnostic expressions (Velupillai et al. 2011; Velupillai 2011). The corpus originates from a medical emergency ward, and specifically text under the heading *Assessment* or *Bedömning* was analysed. In total 3846 documents containing 26,232 sentences were manually annotated and 6483 diagnoses were found. The annotation was carried out by two senior physicians. These diagnoses were annotated for **certainty (positive or negative)**, and **uncertainty (possibly or probably)**, resulting in **six possible certainty levels**: *Certainly Positive, Probably Positive, Possibly Positive, Possibly Negative, Probably Negative* and *Certainly Negative*, see Fig. 4.4.

Levels of Certainty

According to Velupillai (2011) there were, on the negative polarity level, 11% *Certainly Negative* expressions, and 12.2% were in the middle of the scale (*Possibly Positive* and *Possibly Negative*) whilst 47.6% of the expressions were affirmed *Certainly Positive* in the final version of the corpus. The inter- and intra-annotator agreement on the subset that was annotated by both annotators is presented in a confusion matrix in Table 4.4. Velupillai was inspired to use the six different levels

Table 4.4 Confusion matrix, intra- and inter-annotator agreement

	CP	PrP	PoP	PoN	PrN	CN	ND	O	Σ
CP Intra	**990**	78	4	0	3	4	2	19	1100
Inter	***834***	*59*	*7*	*0*	*4*	*5*	*1*	*20*	*930*
PrP Intra	20	**236**	55	1	1	0	1	0	314
Inter	*66*	***134***	*10*	*1*	*0*	*0*	2	*1*	*214*
PoP Intra	4	38	**127**	25	9	0	0	2	205
Inter	*11*	*149*	***180***	*41*	*45*	*1*	*1*	*10*	*438*
PoN Intra	0	0	6	**14**	7	1	0	1	29
Inter	*0*	*0*	*0*	***1***	*5*	*1*	*0*	*0*	*7*
PrN Intra	1	1	1	10	**118**	25	0	5	161
Inter	*0*	*0*	*0*	2	***35***	*18*	*0*	*1*	*56*
CN Intra	2	0	4	0	51	**195**	0	1	253
Inter	2	*0*	*0*	*4*	*99*	***193***	*1*	*3*	*302*
ND Intra	0	0	0	0	0	0	**26**	0	26
Inter	*13*	*5*	*3*	2	*1*	*3*	***30***	*4*	*61*
O Intra	8	1	4	1	7	0	8	**65**	94
Inter	*1*	*1*	*1*	*1*	*5*	*3*	*1*	***49***	*62*
Σ Intra	1025	354	201	51	196	225	37	93	**2182**
Inter	*927*	*348*	*201*	52	*194*	*223*	36	88	**2070**

Table taken from Table 1 in Velupillai et al. (2011) © 2012 with permission from IOS Press. Published in Velupillai et al. (2011)

Columns: Al, first annotation iteration. Rows: Intra: Al, second annotation iteration (same set randomized), Inter: A2. CP = Certainly Positive, PrP = Probably Positive, PoP = Possibly Positive, PoN = Possibly Negative, PrN = Probably Negative, CN = Certainly Negative, ND = Not Diagnosis, O = Other, Σ = Total

by Saurí and Pustejovsky (2009). Saurí and Pustejovsky used a six level scale as well as a label for *Unknown* or *Uncommitted* when they annotated English newswire and broadcast news reports in the FactBank corpus. Their goal was to annotate the degree of factuality of the events.

In Velupillai et al. (2011) the inter-annotator and intra-annotator agreements are presented for the factuality annotations carried out by the two senior physicians. The main finding is that the overall agreement was fairly high (0.7/0.58 F-score and 0.73/0.6 Cohen's κ for intra-/inter- annotator agreement respectively).

Cohen's κ, or Cohen's kappa measures the probability of obtaining high agreement. A kappa value of 0.6 to 0.73 means the task is fairly difficult, indicating that the annotators have moderate to high agreement. A kappa score of 1.0 indicates full agreement (and an easy annotation task). An alternative way of measuring agreement is the F-score, an average result of 0.6–0.7 can be considered quite high. For the whole PhD study about factuality levels in Swedish clinical text see Velupillai (2012).

Negation and Speculations in Other Languages, Such as Chinese

One interesting approach in speculation detection for Chinese clinical notes can be found in Zhang et al. (2016). The authors obtained 0.922 in F-score with a CRF-machine learning approach using 5103 gold-standard speculation annotations as data. One critical point was to obtain a high quality word segmentation to obtain high performance in speculation detection in Chinese, since Chinese does not use spaces as word delimiters.

4.7 Clinical Corpora Available

Generally, it is difficult to get access to clinical corpora for research. This is mainly due to the sensitive information they may contain regarding individuals. We will describe the process of obtaining clinical corpora for research, with ethical permission and de-identification. Most of the few corpora available for research are in English, but some corpora are available in other languages.

4.7.1 English Clinical Corpora Available

The two most well-known clinical corpora are the Informatics for Integrating Biology & the Bedside (i2b2)[3] clinical corpus consisting of approximately 1000

[3]i2b2, http://www.i2b2.org. Accessed 2018-01-11.

notes in English and the Computational Medicine Center (CMC)[4] corpus containing 2216 patient records in American English (Pestian et al. 2007). Another well-used corpora is the Multiparameter Intelligent Monitoring in Intensive Care (MIMIC II)[5] it is also called the De-id corpus and consists of 1934 discharge summaries and 412,509 nursing notes written in American English (Saeed et al. 2011). The BioScope Corpus and the Thyme corpus are two other well-known clinical corpora written in English. The BioScope corpus contains almost 6383 annotated sentences from the clinical domain and is described in Sect. 4.6.2. The Thyme corpus contains 1254 de-identified notes which are annotated for temporal relations. The Thyme corpus is described in Sect. 7.5.5.

The clinical corpora in English are de-identified with respect to sensitive identifiers such as personal names, phone numbers etc. These are identified and removed and some are also pseudonymised, meaning sensitive identifiers are replaced with pseudonyms or surrogates to keep the text natural. This is carried out by using automatic methods combined with manual review of the corpora for residues of sensitive information.

4.7.2 Swedish Clinical Corpora

The Swedish clinical corpora called the Stockholm EPR Corpus contained in the HEALTH BANK—Swedish Health Record Research Bank,[6] from Karolinska University Hospital in Stockholm. It contains over two million patients from over 500 clinical units and encompasses the years 2007–2014. The corpus is de-identified with regard to patient's personal names. Personal identity numbers are replaced with a serial number that makes it possible to follow the patient through the healthcare process, from admission to discharge from the clinical unit (Dalianis et al. 2015).

The Stockholm EPR Corpus contains both structured and unstructured information. The structured data includes gender and age of the patient, admission and discharge date and time, ICD-10 diagnosis codes, drugs both the name and the ATC-codes, blood values, laboratory values etc. The unstructured text consists of physicians' notes and nurses' narratives as well as other notes about the patient from other professionals in the healthcare process.

The Stockholm EPR Corpus is part of the HEALTH BANK—Swedish Health Research Bank. Many smaller subparts of it have been annotated for:

- De-identification, for privacy (Stockholm EPR PHI Corpus).
- and its corresponding Stockholm EPR PHI Pseudo Corpus containing pseudonymised PHI.
- Sentence uncertainty including negations.

---

[4]CMC, https://ncc.cchmc.org/prod/pestianlabdata/request.do. Accessed 2018-01-11.

[5]MIMIC II, http://www.physionet.org/physiotools/deid. Accessed 2018-01-11.

[6]Swedish Health Record Research Bank, http://dsv.su.se/healthbank/. Accessed 2018-01-11.

- Diagnosis factuality, six different levels ranging from affirmative expressions to negations, see Fig. 4.4 for details.
- Clinical (named) entities such as disorders, findings, diagnoses, and body structures and drugs.
- Abbreviations.
- Document classification in two classes, documents containing information on healthcare associated infection or not.
- Adverse drug events (ADE).
  - Attributes, such as negations, speculations, past and future.
  - Relations such as indication, adverse drug event, ADE outcome and ADE cause (these relations will be explained in Sect. 10.2.

All the manual annotations on clinical texts are stored in the HEALTH BANK and are described online.[7] The annotated data is clinical text written in Swedish. The descriptions are in Swedish, but can be understood since the annotation classes are in English and there are numerical values for the number of classes .

4.7.3 *Clinical Corpora in Other Languages than Swedish*

Here follows an enumeration of various clinical corpora in the following languages: Bulgarian, Danish, Dutch, English, Finnish, French, German, Italian, Norwegian, Polish, Spanish, Swedish and Japanese. Many of these corpora are closely connected to individual research groups, and special permission and good contacts are required for access.

- A British English clinical corpus[8] known as the general practice research database used for recognising symptoms automatically. The researchers annotated 6141 records in General Practice/ Primary care (Koeling et al. 2011).
- An Australian English clinical corpus from the Concord hospital's clinical progress summary containing 43,712 anonymised patient records from 2003 to 2008 (Patrick and Nguyen 2011).
- An Australian English pathology corpus from the state of Queensland in Australia containing 45.3 million pathology HL7 messages, including 119,581 histology and cytology reports (Nguyen et al. 2016).
- Another British English clinical corpus containing 20,000 cancer patient records used for semantic annotation and described in Roberts et al. (2009).
- Yet another British English corpus taken from the SLaM BRC Case Register (London area) on 31 December 2014, containing over 250,000 patient records within psychiatry (Perera et al. 2016).

---

[7] Annotated data in HEALTH BANK, http://dsv.su.se/healthbank/annotated-data/. Accessed 2018-01-11.

[8] British English clinical corpus, http://www.gprd.com. Accessed 2018-01-11.

- Another British English corpus is the Health Improvement Network (THIN)[9] database, containing 11 million British English patient records from general practices (Lewis et al. 2007).
- A Bulgarian clinical corpus containing several hundred thousand patient records from the specialties general practice, endocrinology, metabolic disorders cardiology, ophthalmology, gastroenterology, pneumology and physical therapy used for text mining and big data analytics (Boytcheva et al. 2015).
- Another Bulgarian clinical corpus containing 500,000 pseudonymised outpatient records on diabetes (Boytcheva et al. 2017b).
- A Danish clinical corpus containing 61,000 psychiatric hospital patient records from Center for Biological Sequence Analysis (CBS), University of Copenhagen and Technical University of Denmark (Eriksson et al. 2013).
- Another Danish clinical corpus containing 323,122 patient health records used for de-identification (Pantazos et al. 2016).
- A Dutch clinical corpus called the EMC Dutch clinical corpus[10] (Afzal et al. 2014).
- A Finnish clinical corpus[11] containing 2800 sentences from nursing notes from the University of Turku, Finland.
- A French clinical corpus containing 170,000 documents from 2000 patients with a stay of at least 20 days, covering five different hospitals within one geographical area, and several medical specialties (e.g., pneumology, obstetrics, infectious diseases) (Grouin and Névéol 2014).
- Another French clinical corpus containing 59,285 French patient records from three French hospitals. In total the article mentions 115,447 records from six hospitals, including Danish and Bulgarian patient records. The records were used to detect adverse drug events, Chazard et al. (2011).
- Yet another French clinical corpus containing 1500 discharge summaries, half of them containing hospital acquired infections, which are described in Proux et al. (2011).
- A German clinical corpus from Austria, containing 18,000 patient records from eight different clinical units (surgery, vascular surgery, casualty surgery, internal medicine, neurology, anesthesia and intensive care, radiology and physiotherapy) which has been used for document classification (Spat et al. 2008).
- Another German corpus of 12,743 clinical narratives describing laboratory results of leukaemia (Zubke 2017).
- Yet another German corpus of 6817 clinical notes and 118 discharge summaries in nephrology (Roller et al. 2016).
- An Italian clinical corpus containing 23,695 patient records used for entity extraction and determination of semantic relations (Attardi et al. 2015).

---

[9]THIN database, http://www.ucl.ac.uk/pcph/research-groups-themes/thin-pub/database. Accessed 2018-01-11.

[10]EMC Dutch clinical corpus, http://biosemantics.org/index.php/resources/emc-dutch-clinical-corpus. Accessed 2018-01-11.

[11]Finnish clinical corpus, http://bionlp.utu.fi/clinicalcorpus.html. Accessed 2018-01-11.

- A Norwegian clinical corpus containing 7741 patient records encompassing in total 1,133,223 unstructured EHR text documents used for identification of cancer patient trajectories (Jensen et al. 2017).
- A Polish clinical corpus containing 1200 children's hospital discharge records (Marciniak and Mykowiecka 2014).
- A Spanish clinical corpus, the IXAMed corpus from the Galdakao-Usansolo Hospital, collected during 2008–2012 containing 141,800 patient records (Pérez et al. 2017).
- An Argentian-Spanish clinical corpus, containing 512 annotated radiology reports (Cotik et al. 2017).
- A Japanese clinical corpus containing 3012 discharge summaries from the University of Tokyo Hospital annotated for adverse drug events (Aramaki et al. 2010).

For a nice overview of research carried out in clinical text mining in languages other than English see Névéol et al. (2018).

4.8 Summary

Patient record text is different from standard text. Patient records contain plenty of misspellings (up to 10%) and domain specific abbreviations (up to 10%) and acronyms (up to 5%). Patient records also contain incomplete sentences, often the subject or patient is missing in the sentence. In the assessment field there are many negations (up to 10%) since the physician tries to exclude symptoms while reasoning to find the disorder of the patient. In addition to the negations, the content contains vague or uncertain expressions (up to 12%) regarding the factuality of the findings and disorders. Patient record text is written by different professions and also varies between different medical specialties. Discharge summaries are often wellwritten and structured, since they are written for a broader audience than the personnel at the clinical unit. Most available clinical corpora for research are in English; however, there are some corpora in other languages available for research.

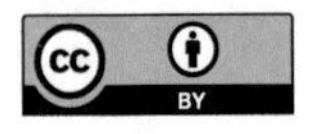

Chapter 5
Medical Classifications and Terminologies

This chapter will present and discuss an important part of clinical text mining, namely the medical classification systems. Medical terminologies, classification systems and available controlled vocabularies are used in healthcare to report, administer, classify and explain diseases and treatment, including medication. In this chapter the history of the medical classification system ICD diagnosis codes will also be told, followed by a description of the more extensive and modern SNOMED CT. For classification of medical literature Medical Subject Headings (MeSH) is used. UMLS developed specifically for mapping between different terminologies and consists of several other terminologies.

ICD-10 is available in several languages, SNOMED CT in some fewer languages and MeSH for even fewer languages. Anatomical Therapeutic Chemical Classification (ATC) codes are used to describe drugs and their chemical components and available in several languages.

We can consider the SNOMED CT and ICD-10 terminologies as the "new" Greek and Latin of medicine. For example, when a ICD-10 diagnosis code such as *J12* is mentioned, everyone knowledgeable in ICD-10 knows that this means the disease *pneumonia* in English, even if the disease is called *lunginflammation* in Swedish.

Other important standards and codes to have knowledge about are *Unstructured Information Management Architecture (UIMA)*, *Fast Healthcare Interoperability Resources (FHIR)*, *Health Level 7 (HL7)* and *OpenEHR*. Many of these classifications have mapping tables between them to perform interoperability. Finally, the matching and mapping of terminologies to clinical text for expanding terminologies will be described.

H. Dalianis, *Clinical Text Mining*, https://doi.org/10.1007/978-3-319-78503-5_5

5.1 International Statistical Classification of Diseases and Related Health Problems (ICD)

ICD stands for *International Statistical Classification of Diseases and Related Health Problems*, but is usually shortened to *International Classification of Diseases*. ICD originates from several early classification systems from the eighteenth century. One is from *Genera morborum*, 1763, the "catalogue of diseases", created by Carl Linnaeus, who is also the father of the classification system for naming organisms. The other source is *Nosologia methodica*, the "disease classification", published by François Boissier de Sauvages de Lacroix in 1763. Linnaeus and Sauvages were good friends and influenced each other.

Significant contributions to the classification of diseases were made by William Farr in 1839, after he was appointed Compiler of Abstracts for the English Registration Act, a law passed on registering the cause of death in the population.

When Florence Nightingale, the social reformer and statistician, and the founder of modern nursing, returned to England from the Crimean War in 1860, she emphasised the importance of a proper statistical classification system for diseases. Jointly with William Farr she worked on the technical problems of the classification system.

Jacques Bertillon was a French physician and statistician who introduced the Bertillon Classification of Causes of Death that is considered to be the predecessor to ICD. Bertillon's system was adopted in 1899 by several countries (Moriyama et al. 2011).

ICD-1, the first revision of the International Statistical Classification of Diseases was published in 1900 (in use 1900–1909): ICD-10, the tenth revision was published in 1986, and has been in use since 1995; however, in the USA they still use ICD-9, the ninth revision.

ICD-10 is the latest revision of ICD-9 and is available in the six official languages of the World Health Organization (WHO), which are Arabic, Chinese, English, French, Russian and Spanish, and in 36 other languages including Swedish. ICD contains 32,000 different diagnosis codes divided into 22 chapters or groups.

ICD coding is used both for medical and administrative purposes. For the clinical personnel to classify diseases and know what type of disease a patient has, but also for administrative purposes such as economical planning and statistics for healthcare.

The 22 chapters are the general foundation, going down to more specific subchapters then more and more specific diseases are observed. For example, the three characters J12 mean *viral pneumonia*[1] at a very basic level. Each three-character level can be extended with up to four characters to provide a more specific definition. The first three characters are separated from the following four characters with a period. This example contains a two-character extension 81, giving J12.81

[1] ICD-10, J12 Viral Pneumonia, http://www.icd10data.com/ICD10CM/Codes/J00-J99/J09-J18/J12-. Accessed 2018-01-11.

- J12 Viral pneumonia, not elsewhere classified
  - J12.0 Adenoviral pneumonia
  - J12.1 Respiratory syncytial virus pneumonia
  - J12.2 Parainfluenza virus pneumonia
  - J12.3 Human metapneumovirus pneumonia
  - J12.8 Other viral pneumonia
    - J12.81 Pneumonia due to SARS-associated coronavirus
    - J12.89 Other viral pneumonia
  - J12.9 Viral pneumonia, unspecified

Fig. 5.1 Hierarchy of the ICD-10 code for J12 Viral pneumonia

which means *pneumonia due to SARS-associated corona virus*; see Fig. 5.1 for the hierarchy of the ICD-10 codes. The final two characters' for the position 6 and 7 signify the increased specificity or lateral position of the disease.

5.1.1 *International Classification of Diseases for Oncology (ICD-O-3)*

There is a special version of ICD, the *International Classification of Diseases for Oncology (ICD-O-3)*,[2] which also is used to code pathology reports for cancer. Pathology reports are also coded using SNOMED CT. ICD-O-3 contains information about the topology and morphology of the cancer. Topology describes the anatomical site of origin, which is where the tumor is situated in the body, and the morphology describes the cell type (histology), stage or behaviour of the tumor (malignant or benign) and number of tumors or metastases.

5.2 Systematized Nomenclature of Medicine: Clinical Terms (SNOMED CT)

SNOMED CT stands for the *Systematized Nomenclature of Medicine-Clinical Terms* and originates from two earlier classification systems called *Systematized Nomenclature of Pathology (SNOP)* from 1965 and the United Kingdom's National Health Service Clinical Terms Version 3 (previously known as the Read Codes). SNOP was created to support American pathologists to classify the pathological observations in the categories etiology, morphology, topography and function. SNOMED CT was released in 2002 (Moriyama et al. 2011).

[2]International Classification of Diseases for Oncology (ICD-O-3), http://codes.iarc.fr. Accessed 2018-01-11.

SNOMED CT is available in US English, UK English, Argentine Spanish, Danish and Swedish. Translations into French, Dutch, Lithuanian and several other languages are underway (IHTSDO 2016). SNOMED CT is a clinical, hierarchical terminology containing medical terms and their relations as well as synonyms, including over 320,000 terms. SNOMED CT contains clinical findings (symptoms), disorders (diagnoses), procedures, body structures, organisms etc. Each concept, description, and relationship has a SNOMED identifier that can have up to 18 digits.

Likewise, if we look at SNOMED CT we can identify the general disorder number 233604007, as the disorder *pneumonia* expressed in English, see Fig. 5.2, where also 35 children or subclasses of pneumonia can be seen. However, it is worth mentioning that physicians still might interpret the ICD-10 codes differently, both intra-language wise and inter-language wise.

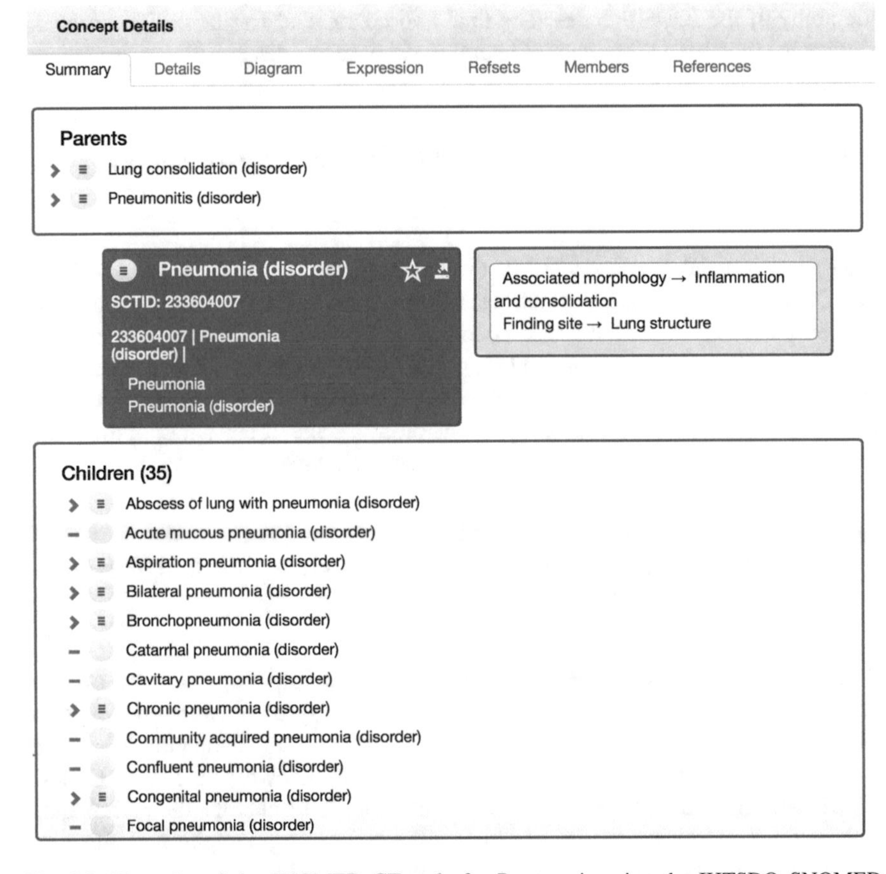

Fig. 5.2 Hierarchy of the SNOMED CT code for Pneumonia using the IHTSDO SNOMED CT Browser (IHTSDO SNOMED CT Browser, http://browser.ihtsdotools.org/?perspective=full&conceptId1=233604007&edition=en-edition&release=v20160731&server=http://browser.ihtsdotools.org/api/snomed&langRefset=900000000000509007. Accessed 2018-01-11)

ICD-10 has a longer history than SNOMED CT and is widely used and well known, while SNOMED CT is less well known. Both terminologies can be used for cross-language information retrieval but also as plain terminologies for various natural language preprocessing steps. In Chap. 10 these preprocessing steps will be described. SNOMED is a hierarchical system with inheritance and is more expressive than ICD-10, but SNOMED is considered to be more difficult to use.

5.3 Medical Subject Headings (MeSH)

MeSH stands for Medical Subject Headings, and is a controlled vocabulary for indexing journal articles and books within life sciences. MeSH was created and is updated by the United States National Library of Medicine (NLM).[3] MeSH is available in over 14 languages.[4]

MeSH is used to categorise publications for libraries, but also to retrieve publications using the MeSH terms. Since MeSH is available in several languages one use cross lingual information retrieval can be used, for example to search in one language and retrieve information in another language.

The 2016 version of MeSH contains in total of 87,000 entry terms (synonyms) to find 27,883 descriptors or subject headings categorised in 16 super headings.[5]

MeSH contains a tree structure from the most general concept to the most specific. If using a MeSH browser different parts of the tree can be browsed, see Fig. 5.3 where the disorder Pneumonia is displayed. The Swedish version of MeSH is a translation of the American-English version, but lacks the amount of synonyms available in English.

5.4 Unified Medical Language Systems (UMLS)

UMLS stands for Unified Medical Language Systems[6] and is only available in English. Its purpose is to support mapping between various terminologies. UMLS contains several million concepts stemming from hundreds of bio(medical) vocabularies, such as ICD-10, MeSH and SNOMED CT as well as medical abbreviations. Liu et al. (2002) extracted 163,666 abbreviations full form pairs from UMLS. To read more about UMLS see Humphreys et al. (1998).

[3]US National Library of Medicine, https://www.nlm.nih.gov/mesh/. Accessed 2018-01-11.

[4]MeSH Translations, https://www.nlm.nih.gov/mesh/MTMS_MeSH.html. Accessed 2018-01-11.

[5]MeSH, https://en.wikipedia.org/wiki/Medical_Subject_Headings. Accessed 2018-01-11.

[6]UMLS, https://www.nlm.nih.gov/research/umls/. Accessed 2018-01-11.

▶ Pneumonia [C08.381.677]
Bronchopneumonia [C08.381.677.127]
Pleuropneumonia [C08.381.677.473]
Pneumonia, Aspiration [C08.381.677.529] +
Pneumonia, Bacterial [C08.381.677.540] +
Pneumonia, Pneumocystis [C08.381.677.675]
Pneumonia, Ventilator-Associated [C08.381.677.800]
Pneumonia, Viral [C08.381.677.807]
Pulmonary Alveolar Proteinosis [C08.381.719]
Pulmonary Atelectasis [C08.381.730] +
Pulmonary Edema [C08.381.742]
Pulmonary Embolism [C08.381.746] +
Pulmonary Eosinophilia [C08.381.750]
Pulmonary Fibrosis [C08.381.765] +
Pulmonary Veno-Occlusive Disease [C08.381.780]
Respiratory Distress Syndrome, Adult [C08.381.840]
Respiratory Distress Syndrome, Newborn [C08.381.842] +
Scimitar Syndrome [C08.381.844]
Solitary Pulmonary Nodule [C08.381.884]
Tuberculosis, Pulmonary [C08.381.922] +

Fig. 5.3 Part of the MeSH tree of Pneumonia. In this example the numerical coding of the MeSH descriptors (MeSH pneumonia entry, https://www.nlm.nih.gov/cgi/mesh/2016/MB_cgi?mode=&term=Pneumonia&field=entry. Accessed 2018-01-11) can be observed

5.5 Anatomical Therapeutic Chemical Classification (ATC)

Each existing drug is represented with an ATC code in the Anatomical Therapeutic Chemical (ATC) Classification[7] which describes each drug with a specific letter and number. The principle of the classification is the active ingredients of the drugs, the organ and structure the act on and their therapeutic, pharmacological and chemical properties. The classification was released in 1976 and is administered by the World Health Organization Collaborating Centre for Drug Statistics Methodology (WHOCC).[8]

ATC codes are structured in five levels. The top level contains the use of the drug, divided in 14 main groups. The second level is the pharmacological and therapeutic subgroup, the third and fourth levels are the chemical, pharmacological and therapeutic subgroups and the fifth level is the chemical substance. The second to fourth levels are used to identify the pharmacological subgroup, see Fig. 5.4 for an example on an ATC code structure.

[7] ATC classification, http://www.whocc.no/atc_ddd_index/.

[8] WHOCC, http://www.whocc.no/atc_ddd_methodology/history/. Accessed 2018-01-11.

A	Alimentary tract and metabolism (1st level, anatomical main group)
A10	Drugs used in diabetes (2nd level, therapeutic subgroup)
A10B	Blood glucose lowering drugs, excl. insulins (3rd level, pharmacological subgroup)
A10BA	Biguanides (4th level, chemical subgroup)
A10BA02	metformin (5th level, chemical substance)

Fig. 5.4 The ATC code structure for the chemical substance *metformin* showing its use in lowering glucose for diabetic patients (ATC, http://www.whocc.no/atc/structure_and_principles/. Accessed 2018-01-11)

Drugs are divided in different groups depending on the chemical substance, their therapeutic effect and their pharmacological group.

5.6 Different Standards for Interoperability

5.6.1 Health Level 7 (HL7)

Health Level 7 (HL7)[9] is the name of a set of standards for the interoperability between different systems in healthcare, for transferring data between patient records systems, and also between patient records systems and laboratory systems or billing systems. See also Health Level Seven International.[10]

Fast Healthcare Interoperability Resources (FHIR)

Fast Healthcare Interoperability Resources (FHIR),[11] is a standard within HL7 for sharing data from an electronic patient record system. FHIR communicates an API via a web interface such as http- and https-protocols, JSON, Cascading Style Sheets and also Java.

[9]HL7, https://en.wikipedia.org/wiki/Health_Level_7. Accessed 2018-01-11.

[10]HL7 International, http://www.hl7.org/. Accessed 2018-01-11.

[11]FHIR, https://en.wikipedia.org/wiki/Fast_Healthcare_Interoperability_Resources. Accessed 2018-01-11.

5.6.2 OpenEHR

OpenEHR[12] is a standard for interoperability specifically between different electronic patient record systems. In Chen and Klein (2007) the open Java interface is described, and in Chen et al. (2009) an experiment performing a bi-directional conversion between the openEHR archetype format to the COSMIC template format is also presented. COSMIC is one of the major electronic patient record systems in Sweden, from Cambio Healthcare Systems. See also the OpenEHR organisation.[13]

UIMA is a special IBM standard for content analytics, see Sect. 8.5.

5.6.3 Mapping and Expanding Terminologies

Medical terminologies and classifications are very useful tools for clinical text mining. They can be used for identifying the semantic meaning of lexical concepts in clinical text. For example, is the concept a disorder, a symptom or a body part? The identification of the semantic meaning can support directly the understanding of the clinical text, but the semantic tagging can also be used as features for machine learning.

One other important use of terminologies is to expand the concept with one or more synonyms. This is valuable for identifying and expanding abbreviations and acronyms in clinical text but also for mapping concepts to other terminologies. However, many of the terminologies and classifications are manually made and do not cover medical subdomains. A shared task in this domain is described in Suominen et al. (2013).

Part of the mapping process is to apply computational linguistic methods such as lemmatisation, stemming and compound splitting, see Sect. 7.3.

To create resources manually for the medical subdomains is time consuming and costly; therefore, unsupervised distributional methods may be used for identifying these concepts. One output of the mapping and expansion task is the creation of synonyms and abbreviation-expansion pairs. A nice overview of the area can be found in Henriksson et al. (2014).

An approach using distributional semantics for identifying abbreviations and synonyms in Swedish clinical text is described in Henriksson et al. (2014), where a combination of two models, Random Indexing and Random Permutation, was used which outperformed a single model. The results measured for recall were 0.39 for abbreviations to expanded forms (long forms), 0.33 for expanded forms (long forms) to abbreviations and 0.47 for synonyms.

[12]OpenEHR, https://en.wikipedia.org/wiki/OpenEHR. Accessed 2018-01-11.

[13]OpenEHR, http://www.openehr.org. Accessed 2018-01-11.

Skeppstedt et al. (2012) used a rule-based approach to match Swedish SNOMED CT terms to a Swedish clinical text. Spelling correction of the clinical text using Levenshtein distance improved the recall slightly.

An approach for Japanese patient blogs is found in Ahltorp et al. (2014) where the authors obtained promising results for the semantic category *pharmaceutical drug* with a recall of 25% for top *n* candidates.

Alfalahi et al. (2015) used an approach utilising distributional semantics implemented as random indexing to find synonyms in Swedish scientific medical text (Läkartidningen). Clustering was used on the semantic vectors to produce centroids. It was shown that the proximity to the centroid of a number of semantically similar seed words was a successful method for ranking candidate terms from the random indexing algorithm.

For more details on abbreviation detection see Sect. 7.3.4.

5.7 Summary of Medical Classifications and Terminologies

This chapter introduced and discussed medical terminologies and standards, the most important being ICD and SNOMED CT specifically used for the patient records but also MeSH for indexing medical literature. ATC classification of drug codes was also introduced; ATC codes describe the chemical components, therapeutic effects and pharmacological class of the drug. All these terminologies and standards are available in several languages.

Different standards for the interoperability of patient record systems were presented. Mapping of terminologies to clinical text was described. The interoperability or mapping of ICD-10 and SNOMED CT will be discussed in Sect. 10.8.8. Other important standards and codes presented were UIMA, FHIR, HL7 and OpenEHR.

Chapter 6
Evaluation Metrics and Evaluation

The area of evaluation of information retrieval and natural language processing systems is complex. It will only be touched on in this chapter. First the scientific base for evaluation of all information retrieval systems, called the Cranfield paradigm will be described. Then different evaluation concepts such as precision, recall, F-score, development, training and evaluation sets and k-fold cross validation will be described. Statistical significance testing will be presented. This chapter will also discuss manual annotation and inter-annotator agreement, annotation tools such as BRAT and the gold standard. An example of a shared task on retrieving information from electronic patient records will be presented.

6.1 Qualitative and Quantitative Evaluation

There are two types of evaluation, *qualitative evaluation* and *quantitative evaluation*. In this book quantitative evaluation is mostly used and described. Qualitative evaluation means asking a user or user groups whether the result from an information retrieval system gives a satisfying answer or not. Qualitative evaluation focuses mostly on one or more users' experiences of a system. Quantitative evaluation means having a mechanical way to quantify the results, in numbers, from an information retrieval system. The Cranfield paradigm will be described, which was the first attempt to make a quantitative evaluation of an information retrieval system.

6.2 The Cranfield Paradigm

The evaluation methods used here are mainly quantitative and are based on the Cranfield tests that also called the *Cranfield Evaluation paradigm or the Cranfield paradigm*, carried out by Cleverdon (1967).

H. Dalianis, *Clinical Text Mining*, https://doi.org/10.1007/978-3-319-78503-5_6

Cyril Cleverdon was a librarian at the College of Aeronautics in Cranfield (later the Cranfield Institute of Technology and Cranfield University), UK. Cleverdon conducted a series of controlled experiments in document retrieval. He used a search device, a set of queries, and test collections of documents and the correct answers. The correct answers consisted of documents answering the questions. These documents are also called relevant documents. The search device had indexed the document collections automatically before the search experiment started.

By using a controlled document collection, a set of controlled queries and knowing the relevant documents, he could run the experiments over and over again after changing different parameters and observe the outcome, measuring precision and recall. Cleverdon proved that single terms taken from the document collection achieved the best retrieval performance in contrast with what he had been trained to do and taught as librarian, which was to perform manual indexing using synonym words from a controlled list.

Voorhees (2001) elaborates on the Cranfield paradigm and argues that this is the only way to evaluate information retrieval systems, since manual objective evaluation is too costly and may be also too imprecise. The Cranfield paradigm has given rise to the Text REtrieval Conference (TREC) and the Cross-Language Evaluation Forum (CLEF), where large controlled document collections together with queries in specific topics are used for the evaluation of information retrieval.

6.3 Metrics

Evaluation, in this case quantitative evaluation, can have many different purposes. There may also be different limitations on the amount data used for training and for evaluation. In some cases, high recall is considered a priority over high precision, and in some cases it is the opposite.

When developing a system, a *development set* is used. A development set is either data for developing rules for an artefact or training material for a machine learning system. In machine learning the development set is often called the *training set* and is used for training the machine learning system. Part of the training set can be put aside for error analysis for the algorithm, and the machine learning algorithm can be adjusted according to the errors, so-called parameter tuning. This part of the training set is called development test set.

A test set is put aside to test the artefact, this test set is neither used for development nor for training and is sometimes called *held out data*, (Pustejovsky and Stubbs 2012).

If data is scarce a method called *k-fold cross validation* is used, this is carried out by dividing the whole dataset into k folds and the k-1 folds are used for training and the remaining one, the 1 fold for evaluation: the folds are switched until all folds are trained and tested on the remaining of the k-1 folds and finally an average is calculated. Usually 10-fold cross validation is used, (Kohavi 1995).

Table 6.1 Confusion matrix: predicted annotation is what the algorithm retrieves or annotates and gold annotation is what was marked up or annotated by a human

		Predicted annotation	
		Positive	Negative
Gold annotation	Positive	True positive (tp)	False negative (fn)
	Negative	False positive (fp)	True negative (tn)

Some false positives that are detected by the algorithm may be correct but wrongly classified by the human annotator (Pustejovsky and Stubbs 2012)

Two metrics used for measuring the performance of a retrieval system are *precision* and *recall*. *Precision* measures the number of correct instances retrieved divided by all retrieved instances, see Formula 6.1. *Recall* measures the number of correct instances retrieved divided by all correct instances, see Formula 6.2. Instances can be entities in a text, or a whole document in a document collection (corpus), that were retrieved. A confusion matrix, see Table 6.1 is often used for explaining the different entities.

Here follow the definitions of precision and recall, see Formulas 6.1 and 6.2 respectively.

$$Precision : P = \frac{tp}{tp + fp} \tag{6.1}$$

$$Recall : R = \frac{tp}{tp + fn} \tag{6.2}$$

The *F-score* is defined as the weighted average of both precision and recall depending on the weight function β, see Formula 6.3. The F_1*-score* means the harmonic mean between precision and recall, see Formula 6.4, when it is written *F-score* it usually means F_1*-score*. The F-score is also called the F-measure. The F_1*-score* can have different indices giving different weights to precision and recall.

$$F\text{-}score : F_\beta = (1 + \beta^2) * \frac{P * R}{\beta^2 * P + R} \tag{6.3}$$

With $\beta = 1$ the standard F-score is obtained, see Formula 6.4.

$$F\text{-}score : F_1 = F = 2 * \frac{P * R}{P + R} \tag{6.4}$$

Precision uses all retrieved documents for the calculation. If there are a large number of documents, there is a possibility to make the calculation simpler by using precision at a cut-off value, for example precision at top 5 or precision at top 10 written as P@5 or P@10 respectively. This measure is called precision at n, or with a general term precision at P@n.

For details on evaluation measurements see Van Rijsbergen (1979), Pustejovsky and Stubbs (2012) and Japkowicz and Shah (2011).

Two evaluation concepts used in medicine and health informatics are *specificity* and *sensitivity*.[1]

- Specificity measures the proportion of negatives that are correctly identified as negative, or not having the condition.
- Sensitivity (the same as recall) measures the proportion of negatives that are correctly identified (e.g., the percentage of healthy people who are correctly identified as not having the condition).

Yet another commonly used metric in medical and clinical systems is *positive predictive value (PPV)* corresponding to precision.

Accuracy is another measurement defined as the proportion of true instances retrieved, both positive and negative, among all instances retrieved. Accuracy is a weighted arithmetic mean of precision and inverse precision. Accuracy can also be high but precision low, meaning the system performs well but the results produced are slightly spread, compare this with hitting the bulls eye meaning both high accuracy and high precision, see Formula 6.5.

$$Accuracy : A = \frac{tp + tn}{tp + tn + fp + fn} \tag{6.5}$$

A *baseline* is usually a value for what a basic system would perform. The baseline system can be a system working in a random way or be a naïve system. The baseline can also be very smart and strong, but the importance of the baseline is to have something to compare with.

If there are other systems using the same data, then it is easy to compare results with these systems and a baseline is not so important.

6.4 Annotation

Annotation in this book means to manually add an annotation to a token or to a set of tokens in text. The reason for this is either to create training material for a machine learning system that uses supervised methods to train, or to create test material to evaluate both machine learning-based tools and rule-based tools. Annotation can also mean to manually classify documents according to predefined classes. *Labelling* is a synonym for annotation.

When performing an annotation task, a decision has to be made on what classes should be annotated and also how to annotate them. Should just the lexical item be

[1]Sensitivity and specificity, https://en.wikipedia.org/wiki/Sensitivity_and_specificity. Accessed 2018-01-11.

annotated or in the case of a personal name, both the first and surname? What about the initial or the title of the person? Likewise when annotating a finding, should the negation modifying the finding be annotated or just the finding? Therefore, guidelines for the annotation task are developed. Usually a couple of test runs of annotations are carried out to test the annotation classes, the settings and the guidelines. The annotators are then allowed to meet and discuss how they reasoned while annotating. After the discussion it is decided how to continue, usually by the chief annotator. New annotation classes are added or redefined and the guidelines are updated (Pustejovsky and Stubbs 2012).

6.5 Inter-Annotator Agreement (IAA)

When annotating data, preferably more than one annotator is used. For finding out the agreement between annotators and the difficulty of the annotation task *inter-annotator agreement (IAA)* is calculated. Inter-annotator agreement is sometimes also called inter-rater agreement. This is usually carried out by calculating the Precision, Recall, F-score and Cohen's kappa, between two annotators. If the IAA is very low, for example an F-score under 0.6, it is considered that the annotation task is difficult, but a low F-score can also be due to the annotators have not been instructed properly on what annotations they should do and the range and format of the annotation or they did not obtain any guidelines. Cohen's kappa measures whether if two annotators might annotate similarly due to chance and not because they agree. Another similar measurement is intra-annotator agreement where the same annotator does his or her task twice on the same text with some time interval to observe the difference between the two sets of annotations, (Pustejovsky and Stubbs 2012).

A gold standard is a manually created set of correct answers, annotations, which is used for evaluation of information retrieval tools, see Sect. 6.8 details.

When building a gold standard usually at least two annotators should agree on the gold standard. Theoretically Cohen's kappa can be used for this task to reveal if the agreement is by chance or not, but for using Cohen's kappa there should not be any variation of number of annotated tokens for each annotator, therefore, F-score is a better measurement between two annotators; however, a high F-score meaning high agreement indicates the task was easy for the annotators.

For document classification there is no variation for length and therefore Cohen's kappa is suitable for statistical significance testing for this task (Artstein and Poesio 2008; Hripcsak and Rothschild 2005; Japkowicz and Shah 2011).

6.6 Confidence and Statistical Significance Testing

The metrics precision and recall can be used to compare the performance of two different algorithms (or classifiers) on a dataset; however, these measurements do not measure if the results found occurred by chance. To confirm that the results are statistically significant *statistical significance testing* has to be carried out.

In Japkowicz and Shah (2011) there is a good overview of statistical significance testing. There any many different statistical methods available to find out if the different results are confident or significant. In this section three methods are going to be described: *McNemar's test*, the *sign test* and *Cohen's kappa* κ.

McNemar's test is commonly used in the case of comparing paired nominal data and specifically the erroneous data to observe if they occur by chance or are errors with some regularity. Produced errors should occur in a regular way, then we know that the results of the classifiers really are different and not by chance, and a conclusion can be drawn on which classifier performs best on this data set. For this to occur the null hypothesis should not be rejected.

McNemar's test is based on the chi-squared (χ^2) test, but while the standard χ^2 test is a test of independence of variables, McNemar's test is for consistency across two variables in a 2×2 contingency table (or misclassification matrix), see Table 6.2.

McNemar's test should only be used if the number of differently classified entities or errors is larger than 20, otherwise the sign test should be used. If there are less than 20 entities the null hypothesis is easily rejected.

To perform the McNemar's Chi-square test with continuity correction use Formula (6.6):

$$\chi^2 = \frac{(|b - c| - 1)^2}{(b + c)} \tag{6.6}$$

where b and c can be found in the contingency table, see Table 6.2.

χ^2 should have a confidence level (P- or probability-value at the χ^2 distribution to not reject the null hypothesis commonly selected P-value is 0.95 with a significance level of 0.05.

The *sign test* is one of the simplest statistical tests. A sign test is a type of binomial test. It can be used to compare two algorithms on multiple domains or multiple data sets. The sign test calculates the number of times one algorithm

Table 6.2 Contingency table describing the output of two algorithms using the same test data giving errors b and c in two cases (Japkowicz and Shah 2011)

		Algorithm 1	
		0	1
Algorithm 2	0	a	b
	1	c	d

0 stands for misclassified and *1* for correctly classified

outperforms the other algorithm on different data sets. The more times one algorithm outperforms the other algorithm, the more confident the results are.

See Japkowicz and Shah (2011) for continued reading on statistical significance testing.

If considering big data, statistical significance testing is not really useful since there is so much data that the results always will be significant!

6.7 Annotation Tools

An *Annotation tool* is a tool for manually annotating of words or text pieces with grammatical categories, named entities, clinical entities etc. There are many different tools that can be used for the annotation work, for a nice review article on annotation tools see Neves and Leser (2012). One commonly used annotation tool is BRAT[2] (Stenetorp et al. 2012).

BRAT runs as a web server on the local computer, and a web browser is used as interface. It is possible to define annotation classes, attributes and relations, and use them for the annotation task. In the specific task shown in Fig. 6.1 a pre-annotation model was trained on annotated records from a medical emergency unit, and was used for the pre-annotation of the records that contain ADE. Observe the complicated *relation arches* for indications, adverse drug reactions and also for the *negated findings* (crossed at), for example "ingen" *andningspåverkan* ("no" respiratory distress). See Sect. 8.2.3 for an explanation of pre-annotation.

6.8 Gold Standard

A *gold standard* is a concept used in information retrieval and natural language processing. A gold standard is a set of correct annotations or correct answers to a query or the correct classification of documents.

A gold standard is created by letting the annotators who have carried out the annotations on the same set decide what the correct annotation is, and agree on this and hence produce a gold standard. There is always a plethora of annotation cases that need to be resolved between annotators, since some annotations are either missing or overlapping. If the annotators cannot agree they may end up with a "silver" standard. Often the chief annotator solve any arguments in the annotation process by making a final decision on the correct answer. There is also a possibility that one of the "best" annotation sets is selected and used as a gold standard.

A gold standard is usually used for evaluation of various developed systems. A gold standard can also be used for training and evaluation of the different systems.

[2]BRAT Rapid Annotation Tool http://brat.nlplab.org/index.html. Accessed 2018-01-11.

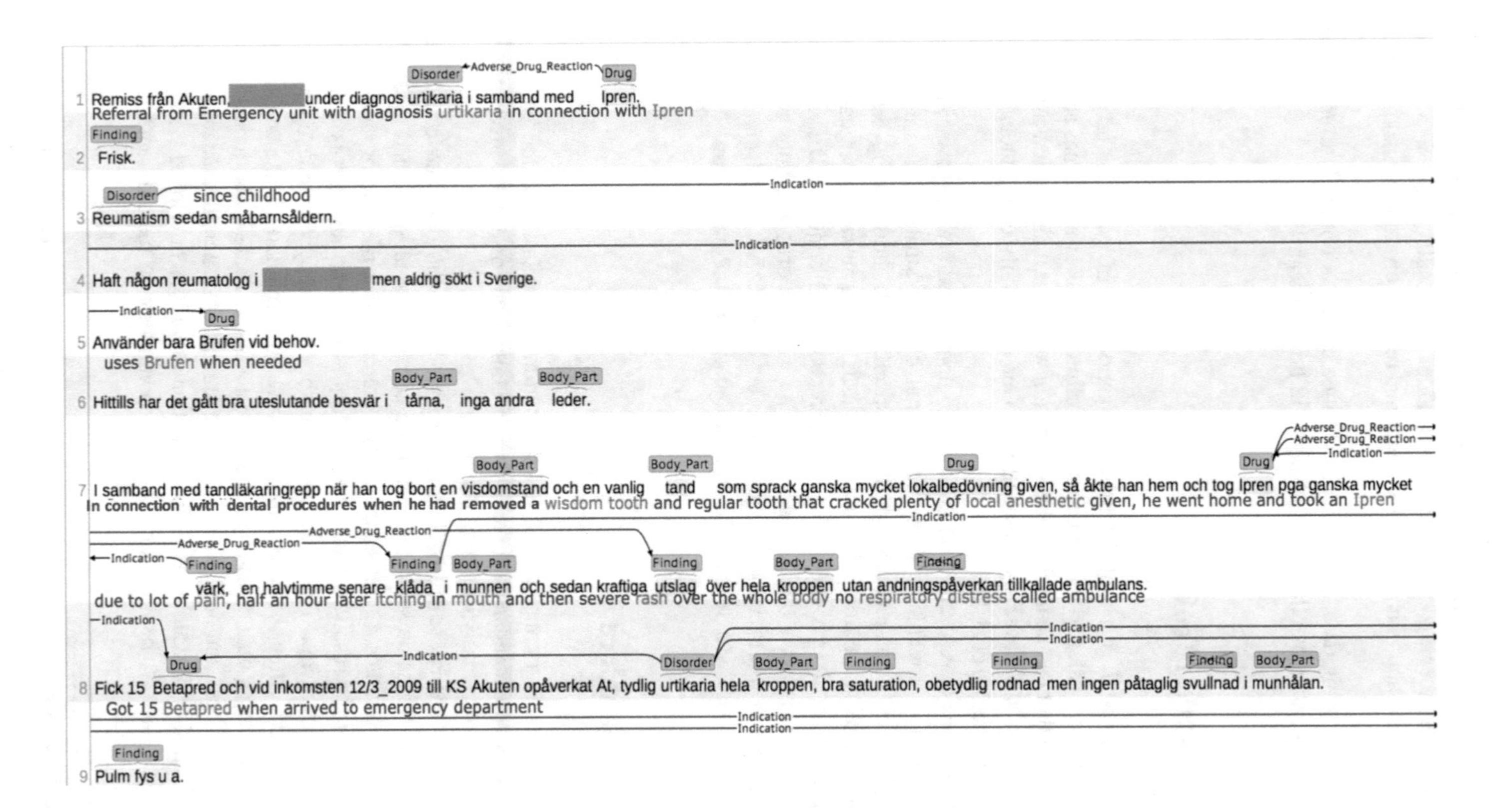

Fig. 6.1 Example of annotation using BRAT on a Swedish (anonymised) clinical text containing an adverse drug event. The example has been manually translated to English

If data is scarce and there is no possibility to divide the gold standard into one development set and a evaluation set, k-fold cross validation can be used instead (Pustejovsky and Stubbs 2012), see Sect. 6.3 on details about k-fold cross validation.

6.9 Summary of Evaluation Metrics and Annotation

This chapter presented evaluation metrics based on the Cranfield paradigm for information retrieval in document collections. Metrics such as precision, recall and F-score were introduced. The concepts development set, and evaluation set and k-fold cross validation were introduced. Manual annotation and inter-annotator agreement were described. The need for statistical significance testing was outlined and various test were presented. Different methods for manual annotations were discussed as well as tools for annotation of clinical text. The concept of the gold standard was introduced.

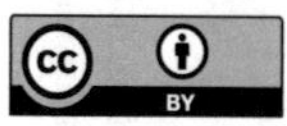

Chapter 7
Basic Building Blocks for Clinical Text Processing

This chapter will describe the basics for text processing and give an overview of standard methods or techniques: Preprocessing of texts such as tokenisation and text segmentation. Word processing such as morphological processing, lemmatisation, stemming, compound splitting, abbreviation detection and expansion. Sentence based methods such as part-of-speech tagging, syntactical analysis or parsing, semantic analysis such as named entity recognition, negation detection, relation extraction, temporal processing and anaphora resolution.

Generally, the same building blocks used for regular texts can also be utilised for clinical text processing. However, clinical texts contain more noise in the form of incomplete sentences, misspelled words and non-standard abbreviations that can make the natural language processing cumbersome. For more details on the concepts in this section, see the following comprehensible textbooks in computational linguistics: Mitkov (2005), Jurafsky and Martin (2014) and Clark et al. (2013).

7.1 Definitions

Natural language processing (NLP) is the traditional term for intelligent text processing where a computer program tries to interpret what is written in natural language text or speech using computational linguistic methods. Other common terms för NLP are computational linguistics, language engineering or language technology.

Information retrieval (IR) may use NLP methods, but the aim with IR is to find a specific document in a document collection, while information extraction (IE) is to find specific information in a document or in a document collection. A popular term today is *text mining*, which means to find previously unknown facts in a text collection or to build a hypothesis that later is to be proven. Text mining is used in a broad sense in the literature sometimes meaning the use of machine learning-based

H. Dalianis, *Clinical Text Mining*, https://doi.org/10.1007/978-3-319-78503-5_7

methods. The term text mining is also used in health informatics mostly meaning the use of rule-based methods to process clinical or biomedical text.

7.2 Segmentation and Tokenisation

Segmentation in NLP is often the first step. It consists of separating sentences from each other (*sentence segmentation*), but also words from each other, (*word segmentation*). Sentences are mostly separated with a period, question mark or comma, but periods and commas may also be used in numerical values; therefore, the segmentation needs to be undertaken carefully.

In Chinese and Japanese separating words from each other is not a trivial task since there are no spaces between words. A word segmenter is therefore needed in these cases.

A text contains a stream of words and other alphanumerical characters, white spaces, interpunctuations and carriage returns, often called *tokens*. *Tokenisation* is the second step for natural language processing. Tokenisation is to decide what a token (or word) is and what should be analysed in the input stream of characters. A tokeniser is therefore needed to extract the tokens in a sentence or text, before performing the "real" natural language processing.

In Fig. 7.1 we can observe a sentence that has been tokenised. There are various choices a tokeniser must take, should sentence delimitaters be included or not? Should constructions such as *let's* be processed in one unit or not? What about the *400* mg/day? How should dosage *mg/day* be tokenised? How about *x-tra*? Usually a standard tokeniser can be used which is built-in in many natural language processing tools. The built-in tokeniser can be adapted to a new domain or a completely new tokeniser can be constructed.

Usually white spaces, sentence delimiters such as commas and question marks, are useful markers for words and can be used as cues for a simple tokeniser. However, clinical text is very noisy and contain many non-standard expressions and the non-standard abbreviations; therefore, tokenisation can be cumbersome.

In the article by Patrick and Nguyen (2011), the authors explain the problems with tokenisation of clinical text nicely and also show how to solve parts of it. They give an example of *HR 72*, consisting of both an acronym for heart rate measurement

The patient has signs of tuberculosis in his left lung, let's try a new treatment with x-tra Isoniazid, 400 mg/day.

This sentence is tokenised as

"The" "patient" "has" "signs" "of" "tuberculosis" "in" "his" "left" "lung" "," "let" "'" "s" "try" "a" "new" "treatment" "with" "x" "-" "tra" "Isoniazid" "," "400" "mg" "/" "day" "."

Fig. 7.1 Example of a sentence in a clinical text and its tokenisation

and the value of *72*, which need to be treated as one unit *heart rate 72*. Typically also dates such as *3/7/02*, need to be treated as single units.

7.3 Morphological Processing

The next step is morphological processing of each token. Morphological processing is to analyse the morphemes of the words, the different parts as inflections both such as prefixes, infixes or suffixes. Some of the tokens form multiword expressions, that is two or more consecutive tokens which should be processed jointly, for example *heart rate*. Clinical text also contains combinations of abbreviations and full forms making the morphological processing difficult.

7.3.1 Lemmatisation

Lemmatisation is the process of finding the base form of a word. It is specifically useful for inflected languages, such as German, Polish, Russian, Swedish etc. English is on the contrary a language with simple morphology and does need very advanced lemmatisation. The lemmatisater will process the words to their base form or lemma. Lemmatisation makes the variation of the same word with different inflection less frequent, by collapsing the different inflected forms of the same word into one lemma, and makes it easier in many natural language processing systems to process words and also their meaning. There are many different off-the-shelf lemmatisers available to use. Lemmatisers are often built-in in taggers, that decides on the word class or function of a word, see Sect. 7.3.6.

Regarding inflected languages such as Swedish and German, many meaning bearing words such as nouns are inflected, both in plural but also in determined or undetermined form. In German the four noun cases affect the inflection of the noun. Therefore, these should be *lemmatised*, to obtain the base or lemma form.

7.3.2 Stemming

A *stemmer* can sometimes be used instead of a lemmatiser. A stemmer is a more basic or raw form of lemmatisation. A stemmer performs stemming on the word and reduces the word to a stem, which may not be a real word (lemma) but a representation of the word. For example, the inflected words *pathology, pathologies, pathological* and *pathologically* can be stemmed to *pathology*, which actually happens to be real word.

Useful stemmers are found in the Snowball system[1] available on GitHub. The GitHub website for the Snowball stemmer also contains a set of stop word lists for different languages that can be used for preprocessing of corpora. Stop words are non-functional words such as *and, or, in, on, also, with* etc., usually these are high frequency words constituting approximately 40% of the words in a text. There are usually around 200 typical stop words in each language.

Stemming usually increases recall and decreases precision in a retrieval setting, but not always, it may also increase precision (Carlberger et al. 2001).

7.3.3 Compound Splitting (Decompounding)

In compounding languages, such as Swedish and German, some of the tokens should be decompounded and eventually processed to their base form. Compound splitting or decompounding is performed using dictionaries, in combination with rules for decompounding.

For example, in Swedish *diabetespatient* "patient with diabetes" should be decompounded to *diabetes patient*, or the plural form *diabetespatienter* "patients with diabetes" should be decompounded to *diabetes patienter*. The decompounded plural form can then be lemmatised to *diabetes patient*. As *diabetes* is in its base form already the lemmatiser does not need to do anything, but *patienter* is in its plural form and needs lemmatisation to *patient*, its lemma form.

Abbreviations can be compounds of regular words and abbreviations, as in the Swedish clinical abbreviation *lungrtg* meaning *lungröntgen* (chest X-ray). The equivalent in English is *chestx* meaning *chest X-ray*. To perform compound splitting or decompounding one needs dictionaries, and also rules for compounding words. Another issue is how far the decompounding should be carried out not to remove the meaning of the word so it becomes meaningless.

A decompounder for Swedish medical words can be found on the DSV website.[2]

7.3.4 Abbreviation Detection and Expansion

Clinical text contains a proportion of abbreviations ranging from 3% to 10% of the total text, see Sect. 4.4. Many of the abbreviations, up to 33%, are ambiguous; therefore, they need to be disambiguated.

To process abbreviations first they need to be detected and then expanded (or normalised). There have been some studies to solve this. One approach for English

[1] Snowball system, http://snowballstem.org. Accessed 2018-01-11.

[2] Medical Decompounder for Swedish, http://dsv.su.se/en/research/research-areas/health/medical-decompounder-for-swedish. Accessed 2018-01-11.

clinical text was carried out by Xu et al. (2007). One simple method used to detect abbreviations was to match them to dictionaries, both standard and medical dictionaries and taking into account morphological variants of the words. The words that did not give any match were either possible abbreviations or possible misspellings.

Another method is an *heuristic* (or *rule of thumb*) rule-based method based on the form of abbreviations in clinical text, for example words fulfilling one of the following criteria (Xu et al. 2007):

1. If the word contains any special characters such as hyphen "-" or a period ".".
2. If the word contains less than six characters and also contains:
   (a) a mixture of alphabetic and numeric characters.
   (b) capital letter(s), but not followed by a period or first capital letters.
   (c) words with lower case letters, but not contained in any word list.

For Swedish, Isenius et al. (2012) used similar heuristic rule-based methods as Xu et al. (2007) in their prototype *SCAN: A Swedish clinical abbreviation normalizer* to detect abbreviations utilising common abbreviation patterns such as hyphenations etc., but they also decided to check words with a length from three to eight characters as possible abbreviations. The performance of the heuristic rule-based method was measured to a precision of 81% and a recall of 76%, evaluated on 2050 abbreviations in a clinical text manually annotated by a senior physician.

SCAN was developed further for the detection and expansion of abbreviations in clinical text. SCAN obtained an F-score of 0.85 for detection of abbreviations in assessment entries from an emergency department and an F-score 0.83 for detection of abbreviations in radiology notes from a radiology department. Regarding expansions of abbreviations, SCAN obtained 79% correct expansions for the assessment entries and 61% correct expansions for the radiology notes. A set of abbreviation lexicons for Swedish clinical text was created and is available on the DSV website.[3] They are in the form of the abbreviation and the expanded abbreviation (Kvist and Velupillai 2014).

For abbreviation expansion and synonym extraction for Swedish, Henriksson et al. (2014) used a combination of two distributional models Random Indexing and Random Permutation, applied both to a Swedish clinical corpus and also to Swedish medical scientific corpus, *Läkartidningen*. The best results were obtained for a combination of semantic spaces originating from a single corpus. The best results for a list of ten candidate terms, measured in recall, were for the following three tasks: Abbreviations to long forms gave 39% recall, and for long forms to abbreviations gave 33% recall, when evaluating two different terminologies containing these terms.

Tengstrand et al. (2014) also used a distributional semantic approach but combined it with Levenshtein distance to choose the correct candidate among seman-

[3] Swedish Medical Abbreviations, http://dsv.su.se/en/research/research-areas/health/swedish-medical-abbreviations. Accessed 2018-01-11.

tically related words. The domain was Swedish radiology reports and Swedish scientific medical text *Läkartidningen*. Filtering and normalisation with Levenshtein distance gave an improvement of 22% compared with only using distributional semantics which gave correct expansion of the abbreviation in 40% of the cases.

There was also a shared task as part of the ShARe/CLEF eHealth Challenge 2013 to detect and expand abbreviations and acronyms (which the authors called normalising) to aid patients understanding of clinical text, as described in Mowery et al. (2016). The results were state of the art, but acronyms and abbreviations with high ambiguity and two or more meanings were particularly challenging for the normalisation systems.

A Machine Learning Approach for Abbreviation Detection

Xu et al. (2007) also used a machine learning-based method for abbreviation detection. The features used were the same as in their rule-based method. The best results were obtained when using the machine learning algorithm j48 decision tree in the Weka toolkit, extended with external resources from UMLS as well as the average document frequency of a word in the analysed clinical text, giving a precision of 91.4% and a recall of 80.3%.

Wu et al. (2011) used the machine learning algorithm Random Forest trained on 1386 annotated abbreviations in a small English clinical corpora, containing in total 18,225 tokens. The authors obtained an F-score of 0.948, a precision 98.8% and recall of 91.2%.

Regarding expansion or normalisation of abbreviations found in clinical text, Wong et al. (2006) describe a method where they use a combination of an abbreviation dictionary and the Aspell spelling correction algorithm that makes suggestions on possible expansions.

Zeng et al. (2012) used topic models trained on English clinical text to expand queries for an information retrieval task, their topic model approach improved F-score and recall by up to 0.38, but decreased precision when compared with the baseline method.

For more on expansion of terminologies see Sect. 5.6.3.

7.3.5 Spell Checking and Spelling Error Correction

Spell checkers consist of two parts *spell checking* and *spelling error correction*. Spell checking, or spelling error detection is the process to find out if a word is misspelled, if it is misspelled it can then be corrected. This can be done by performing lemmatisation on the inflected word, and matching the lemma to a dictionary to confirm the spelling.

To correct the misspellings the *Damerau–Levenshtein distance*, also called edit error distance, or just edit distance, can be used. Common errors can be corrected using the following four edit errors operations: *insert, delete, substitute* or *transpose*. Each operation changes a single character in a string and the number of operations is counted. The minimal number of operations is counted until a correct match is obtained with the corresponding word in the dictionary. These four operations cover almost 80% of the possible human-made misspellings performed using a keyboard. The edit distance for a misspelled word rarely exceeds two operations.

The Damerau–Levenshtein distance is sometimes called The Levenshtein distance, but then the *transpose* operation is excluded (Damerau 1964; Levenshtein 1966).

Soundex is an older phonetic spelling algorithm used to match words as they are pronounced in English, homophones are encoded similarly so they can be matched. The Soundex algorithm was used mainly for matching similar spelling of names. Kukich (1992) has written a good overview of the spelling correction area.

The next step after spelling error correction is grammar correction, but it will not be discussed in this book since, to our knowledge, it has not yet been carried out for clinical text.

Spell Checking of Clinical Text

Wong and Glance (2011) normalised noisy English clinical progress notes. These contained both misspellings and abbreviations. The authors used web data as a dictionary for their spelling error correction system, together with statistical information derived from the web including the distributional behaviour or what the authors call statistical semantics. The system also calls on the occasional interaction of clinicians, and the system learns and improves from the human interaction. The spelling error correction system obtained 88.73% accuracy.

Ruch et al. (2003) constructed a spelling error correction system for French clinical records. The system is organised in three modules: The first module is a standard context-independent spell checker. The second module tries to rank the candidates from the first module using morpho-syntactic disambiguation tools (part-of-speech tools (POS)) and the third module processes words using the same part-of-speech (POS) tools and word-sense (WS) disambiguation. Finally, as one more improvement the authors added a named entity recogniser to avoid correcting named entities that cause many correction errors. The authors obtained 95% correction of spelling errors.

Siklósi et al. (2016) presented a context-aware system based on statistical machine translation (SMT) to correct spelling errors in Hungarian clinical text. The authors did not have access to any word list with correctly spelled clinical terms or to parallel corpora with correct and misspelled clinical text, so they used SMT as support to select possible correctly spelled candidate terms. The SMT system assisted in choosing possible context where the term was correctly spelled. The SMT with language model from the medical domain obtained an accuracy of 87.23%.

Grigonyte et al. (2014) developed an approach to detect and correct spelling errors in Swedish clinical text. Since many clinical misspellings are a combination of abbreviations and misspellings, the authors used abbreviation detection combined with lexical normalisation of compounds and misspellings. This spelling error correction approach reached 83.9% precision and 76.2% recall.

The Hunspell spelling system is adapted to languages with rich morphology, and was originally developed for Hungarian. In OpenOffice.org Hunspell supports over 98 languages (Pirinen and Lindén 2010). When using these spell checkers for clinical text medical, or clinical dictionaries need to be added, see Patrick and Nguyen (2011).

Patrick and Nguyen (2011) wrote a nice overview over different studies to create a clinical text spell checking and correction system. In the same article the authors describe the use of SNOMED CT for English as a dictionary for the spelling correction algorithm, matching the SNOMED CT descriptions to clinical text for assigning codes. Using the spelling correction increased the SNOMED CT coded content of 15% and the number unique codes increased by 4.7%.

An approach for spelling error correction of Swedish clinical text was performed by Dziadek et al. (2017), where the authors used the Swedish version of SNOMED CT, MeSH, ICD-10 and NSL[4] as dictionaries for checking the correctness. The study tried out several spelling error correction methods such as Levenshtein threshold, a context-sensitive method based on trigram frequencies and a corpus-based dictionary. The corpus-based dictionary contains words that occur more than twice. Of the detected misspellings, a subset of 571 were manually evaluated by a senior physician, she categorised 222 of these as misspelled. Of the 222 misspellings, 70% were correctly edited by the algorithm. (Note that clinical text contains around 10% misspellings).

A lower Levenshtein threshold gave both higher spelling error correction and mapping precision, while a higher Levenshtein threshold gave more SNOMED mappings.

For details on the approach see the master's thesis of Dziadek (2015)

Open Source Spell Checkers

There are a number of open source spell checkers to use, for example Aspell or Hunspell,[5] often with dictionaries for different languages, to use them in the medical domain specific dictionaries need to be added or created.

[4]The Swedish National Substance Register for Medicinal Products maintained by the Medical Products Agency—Läkemedelsverket.

[5]Hunspell, http://hunspell.github.io. Accessed 2018-01-11.

There is a specific Swedish spell checking system called Stava[6] which can be used for spell checking PDF, HTML, LaTeX and DOC-format documents. Stava is open source and can be downloaded freely.[7]

For a general English spell checker see an implementation in Python of Peter Norvig's spell checker[8] by Nick Sweeting in 2014.

Regarding grammar checkers for clinical text, nothing has so far been reported in academic literature.

Search Engines and Spell Checking

One interesting point is that search engines do not use general dictionaries to perform spell checking on the search questions but uses the index as a dictionary. This means all words contained in the document collection or corpora are indexed and available as a dictionary. The search engine will then propose correct words that are in the document collection to assist the user to find what he or she is looking for. There is no point for the search engine in proposing correctly spelled words that are not available in the document collection.

7.3.6 Part-of-Speech Tagging (POS Tagging)

The next step of the NLP pipeline is *part-of-speech tagging*, which is the process of automatically extracting the function of the words: *determiner, subject, predicate, adjective, adverb, preposition* etc. There are also other types of tagging, such as semantic or thematic tagging.

Each word is usually classified in a word class, such as *noun, adjective, adverb, determiner* and *preposition*, but when analysing a sentence, the words have functions depending on how they relate to each other, for example: *subject, predicate, direct object* and *indirect object*, this is what a part-of-speech tagger will determine.

There are several methods for constructing taggers, both rule- or dictionary based, but machine learning approaches are state of the art. There are several taggers available for use, one tagger for each language, or at least one tagger and one

[6]Stava, (interface in Swedish), http://www.csc.kth.se/stava. Accessed 2018-01-11.

[7]Stava download (in Swedish), http://www.nada.kth.se/~viggo/stava/manual.php. Accessed 2018-01-11.

[8]Peter Norvig's spell checker in Python, https://github.com/pirate/spellchecker. Accessed 2018-01-11.

language model for each language to tag.[9] For English we have, for example, the TnT tagger, which can be trained on manually annotated corpora. For Swedish we have the Granska tagger and Stagger—the Stockholm Tagger.

7.4 Syntactical Analysis

Syntactical analysis or *parsing* is the next step, to find the syntactical structure of a sentence. The syntax determines the order of the lexical items in a sentence. To do so, a grammar describing the language according to the order in which words occur in a sentence is needed. Usually there are grammar rules describing the language and a parser executes the grammar rules. Sentence grammar describes the sentences but also phrases constituting the whole sentence. A text grammar is used for describing a whole text, which constitutes a set of sentences.

Previously, linguists constructed rules manually, usually several thousand rules were necessary to parse natural language correctly. Today, manually annotated text is used as data to train machine learning systems on the behaviour of the language to produce the grammar rules automatically. The grammar model is then used to parse a text. Of course a parser will also use information from a tagger to carry out the parsing.

A parser can work bottom-up, top-down or incrementally with noisy text, or backtracking, left to right, dependency-based etc. The output from a parser is a syntactic tree describing the different parts of the sentence.

The textbook in natural language processing by Jurafsky and Martin (2014) gives a good description of the available parser methods.

One possible parser to use is MaltParser, which is a dependency-based parser.[10] MaltParser has pre-trained models for Swedish, English, French and Spanish (Nivre et al. 2006).

Hassel et al. (2011) used MaltParser with a pre-trained model for Swedish and applied it on Swedish clinical text, they obtained comparably good result for part-of-speech tagging with an accuracy of 92.4%. This result should be considered in the context of clinical text, which is very noisy and in a completely different domain than the pre-trained model of the MaltParser was trained on. Observe also MaltParser needs as input text that has been morphosyntactically disambiguated using a tagger. In Fig. 7.2 we can see the dependency tree from the parsing of a clinical text.

[9] Part-of-speech taggers, https://en.wikipedia.org/wiki/Part-of-speech_tagging#External_links. Accessed 2018-01-11.

[10] MaltParser, http://www.maltparser.org. Accessed 2018-01-11.

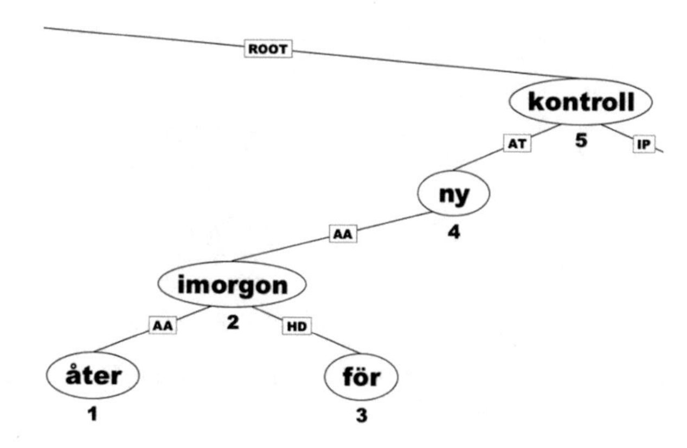

Fig. 7.2 Example dependency parse tree for the Swedish sentence *åter imorgon för ny kontroll* ("back tomorrow for new check-up") from MaltParser (© 2011 Northern European Association for Language Technology (NEALT). Reprinted with the permission of NEALT and the authors. Published in Hassel et al. 2011)

Another useful parser supporting the standard for universal dependencies[11] is the UD-parser[12] that supports over 50 languages (Nivre et al. 2016). The UD-parser is a variant of MaltParser.

7.4.1 Shallow Parsing (Chunking)

A more basic form of parsing is shallow parsing. Shallow parsing (also called chunking, or "light parsing") is something between POS tagging and parsing. The shallow parser or chunker detects constituent parts in sentences in the form of nominal phrases or verb phrases.

7.4.2 Grammar Tools

There are many tools to create grammars. Grammars are used to parse text, or in other words to syntactically analyse text. One such grammar is the definite clause grammar (DCG) form, implemented in the *Prolog* logic programming language. In DCG a grammar can be written in an abstract form and be compiled to an executable Prolog form, see Fig. 7.3. Prolog was constructed in 1972 and was originally created for natural language processing.

[11] Universal Dependencies v2, http://universaldependencies.org. Accessed 2018-01-11.

[12] UDPipe, https://ufal.mff.cuni.cz/udpipe. Accessed 2018-01-11.

```
sentence --> noun_phrase, verb_phrase.
noun_phrase --> det, noun.
verb_phrase --> verb, noun_phrase.
det --> [the].
det --> [a].
noun --> [cat].
noun --> [bat].
verb --> [eats].
```

Fig. 7.3 Example of a toy DCG in Prolog, that can parse the sentence: *The cat eats the bat*, and some variations on this, (from Wikipedia)

The DCG-grammar (and Prolog) can be considered as a set of theorems and the lexical items as facts that have to be proved by using a theorem prover. The theorem prover is the built-in Prolog interpreter. If the facts (the lexical items), in the theorems (the grammar) are proved, corresponding to that the syntax of the tested sentence is correct. One more advantage of DCG is that it can easily be extended to produce a syntax tree that can be used to perform operations on. The DCG is very similar to the *Backus-Naur Form (BNF)* for writing grammars.

Other tools originally developed for building compilers for formal languages, such as programming language is *Lex (Lexical Analysis)* and *Yacc (Yet another compiler-compiler)*,[13] which both are built-in in the Linux operating system. These can also be used to construct parsing tools for natural languages.

7.5 Semantic Analysis and Concept Extraction

Semantic analysis is the task of interpreting the meaning or semantics of entities that were identified. Semantic analysis is also called text analytics. There are several ways to do semantic analysis. One is to analyse the syntactic parse tree and to assign parts of it meaning. Traditionally predicate logic has been used as a representation, but there are many other representations. Other simpler tasks are named entity recognition and negation detection along with more complex tasks such as factuality or uncertainty detection tasks. Relations extraction and temporal processing are also complex semantic tasks as well as anaphora resolution. All these tasks are going to be discussed in the following subsections.

[13]Lex and Yacc page, http://dinosaur.compilertools.net. Accessed 2018-01-11.

7.5.1 *Named Entity Recognition*

Named Entity Recognition (NER) or Named Entity Tagging was first defined in the MUC 7 challenge as the identification of *personal names, locations, organisations* and *time points* or *dates*, also called TIMEX expressions in newswire text (Chinchor and Robinson 1997), but now it has broadened to include almost anything interesting in a text. In clinical text NER usually means the named entities for de-identifying text, such as *personal names, addresses* and *telephone numbers* etc but also *finding (symptom), disorder (disease), drug* and *body part* when referring to *clinical (named) entity mining*.

To perform NER, traditionally, name lists or so-called Gazetteers, have been used combined with regular expressions: today most of the approaches use machine learning techniques, except for extracting numerical expressions, such as telephone numbers or drug dosages, where regular expressions are more efficient.

Machine Learning for Named Entity Recognition

In the study by Skeppstedt et al. (2014) patient records from a Swedish internal medicine emergency unit were annotated with the named entities *disorder, finding, pharmaceutical drug* and *body structure* by two senior physicians. The inter-annotator agreement (IAA), was calculated to an F-score of 0.77 for disorder, 0.58 for finding, 0.88 for pharmaceutical drug and 0.80 for body structure. The annotated corpus is called the *Stockholm EPR Clinical Entity Corpus*.

A number of features were extracted for the training data. The features were based on the terminology in ICD-10 diagnosis codes, SNOMED CT and MeSH as well as on pharmaceutical drugs from the Swedish FASS,[14] but also on POS tagging and lemmatisation of the input words.

The features were extracted by matching each token from the training text with tokens in the ICD-10, SNOMED CT, MeSH or pharmaceutical drugs description text. These features, the manual annotated data, and all tokens were used as training data utilising the implementation CRF++ of the Conditional Random Fields algorithm. The best results for CRF++ were obtained for lemmas, POS tags and terminology matching for the current token and the previous token as well as compound splitting for the current token. This final model obtained an F-score of 0.81 for disorder, 0.69 for finding, 0.88 for pharmaceutical drug, 0.85 for body structure and 0.78 for the combined category disorder + finding. These results are compared with other researchers' results on clinical texts in Fig. 7.4. Both rule-based and machine learning-based approaches were used.

The system by Skeppstedt et al. (2014) is called *Clinical Entity Finder (CEF)* and has been used as a *pre-annotation system* in Henriksson et al. (2015). In Fig. 7.4 we

[14]Farmaceutiska Specialiteter i Sverige (FASS) is the Swedish version of the American Physician's Desk Reference.

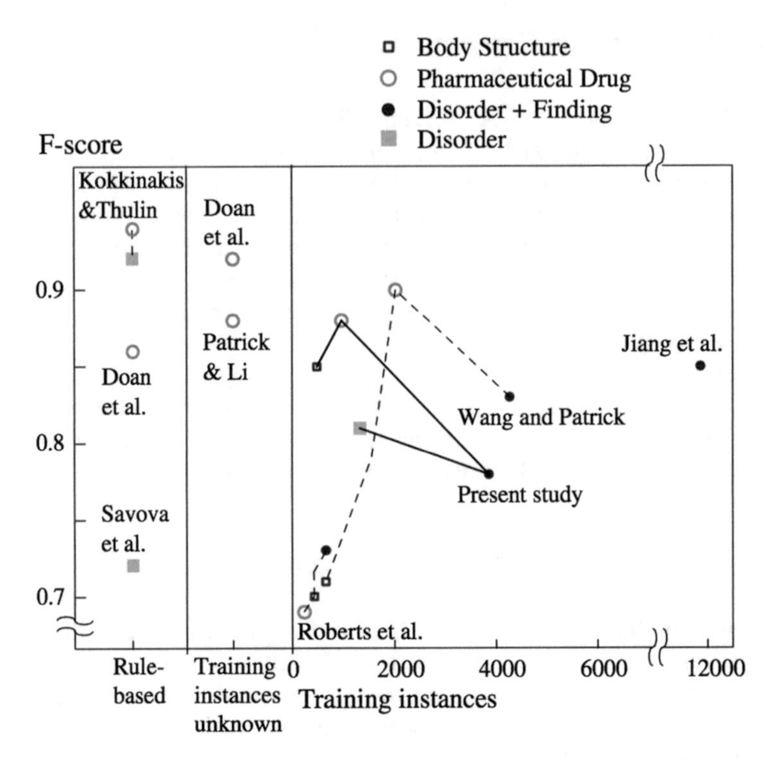

Fig. 7.4 Diagram of clinical entity recognition systems: *Comparison to a number of previous clinical NER studies. Results from the same studies are connected with a line: a solid line for the present study and dashed lines for previous studies. The first column from the left shows the result of three rule-base studies, and the second column shows the result of two machine learning studies for which the number of used training instances were not reported. The rest of the diagram shows the result of a number of machine learning studies for which the number of training instances were reported. The entity names of the present study are used for denoting comparable entity types in previous studies.* Diagram and text cited from Skeppstedt et al. (2014). Present study is the study by Skeppstedt et al. (2014) (© 2014 Elsevier Inc. All rights reserved-reprinted with permission from Elsevier Inc. Published in Skeppstedt et al. 2014)

can see the results compared to other researchers' result. Regarding pre-annotation see Sect. 8.2.2.

In the 2010 i2b2/VA challenge on concepts, assertions and relations in clinical text (Uzuner et al. 2011), there is a nice overview of both entity and relation detection of clinical concepts. The best assertion extraction or clinical named entity recognition system used Conditional Random Fields (CRF) and obtained an F-score of around 0.90.

Regarding medication identification such as *drug names, brand names, dosages, modes, frequencies* and *reason*, there was a *2010 i2b medication challenge*, (Uzuner et al. 2010). Twenty teams participated in the challenge; the ten rule-based approaches scored best; however, the best performing system was hybrid-based. The best performing hybrid system used the machine learning algorithms CRF and

SVM to detect clinical entities, and pattern matching rules to determine whether two entities were related and to detect negations.

Regarding various studies on both rule-based and machine learning-based clinical entity recognition, the PhD thesis by Skeppstedt (2015) is a good place start.

7.5.2 Negation Detection

Negation detection in clinical text mining is the task to detect negations that modify the clinical entities that are affirmed, for example findings, disorders, body parts and drugs. The negation of clinical entities, such as affirmed symptoms and diagnoses, makes them not valid, for example *no cough* or *no fever*. Negation can also be considered as a special case of factuality detection where negation is the weakest factuality consequently pure negation, or that the fact is not valid since it is negated.

Negation Detection Systems

One of the earliest approaches of detecting negations was the construction of *NegEx*. NegEx is a simple regular expression algorithm. NegEx uses three different negation trigger lists and one list containing finding and disorder. The contents of these lists are matched to the input clinical text string to decide if a concept (finding and disorder) in the string is negated or not (Chapman et al. 2001).

Negation Trigger Lists

The first trigger list in NegEx is called the pre-negation list and contains possible trigger phrases, that should be found before the negated word, for example the phrase *no signs of*. The second trigger list is called the post-negation list and contains a possible trigger phrases that should be found after the negated word, such as *unlikely*. Finally, the third trigger list contains possible pseudo-negations, they look like negation triggers but are not, for example *not certain if*.

The contents of these negation triggers are matched to the input text string and when a negation is found the distance is calculated in the form of the number of words from the negation. The distance to the negation should be in the maximum range of six words from the finding or a disorder (disease) in the input string. The list of the findings or the disorders is based on findings and disorders from UMLS.

The original English version of NegEx obtained a precision of 84.5% and a recall of 82.4% when tested on discharge summaries.

Later NegEx was extended to a version called ConText (Harkema et al. 2009) that also detected historical, hypothetical and related persons condition.

NegEx for Swedish

Skeppstedt (2011) adapted the rule-based NegEx to Swedish. The Swedish version of NegEx obtained a precision of 75.2% and a recall of 81.9%, evaluated on the assessment field from randomly chosen Swedish patient records from the Stockholm EPR Corpus. Hence the English version obtained better results than the Swedish version, but the English version was evaluated on a different corpus and language.

Negation trigger list for English[15] and for Swedish[16] can be found online.

NegEx for French, Spanish and German

NegEx was adapted to French by Grouin et al. (2011), the authors also extended NegEx to treat conjunctions and possible negations by adding two more trigger lists. The French NegEx obtained an F-score of 0.863 when evaluated. NegEx was also ported to Spanish, by Costumero et al. (2014), they obtained an accuracy of 84.8%, and also ported to German obtaining an F-score of 0.9 (Cotik et al. 2016).

In an approach by Chapman et al. (2013) the English NegEx was extended to Swedish, French and German and compared. The negation triggers *no* and *not* were similar for all languages. French had the largest diversity on triggers, while German had the least diversity. Agglutination in Swedish and German causes problems for example in Swedish *diabetesfri* means *(diabetes free)*, hence *ej diabetesfri,* means *(has diabetes)*, this can not be processed by NegEx. French negations are inflected depending on gender and number agreement, making it difficult to construct trigger lists.

Machine Learning Approaches for Negation Detection

In a machine learning approach, annotated corpora of Swedish and English negation cues were used as training and evaluation data for the Stanford NER which is based on Conditional Random Fields (CRF) algorithm. The Swedish corpus Stockholm

[15]NegEx trigger list for English, https://github.com/chapmanbe/negex/blob/master/genConText/negex_triggers.txt. Accessed 2018-01-11.

[16]NegEx trigger list for Swedish, http://people.dsv.su.se/~mariask/resources/triggers.txt. Accessed 2018-01-11.

EPR Sentence Uncertainty Corpus (Dalianis and Velupillai 2010a), and the English corpus the BioScope corpus (Vincze et al. 2008) were used. Both corpora were annotated for negations and uncertainty. For Swedish a precision of 87.9% and a recall of 91.7% was obtained for negation cues. For English a precision of 97.6% and a recall of 96.7% was obtained for negation cues. A possible explanation for the better results for English is that the English BioScope corpus is a better and more thoroughly annotated corpora.

Other approaches for detecting negated expressions in English clinical text were investigated by Huang and Lowe (2007), the authors used both parse trees and regular expressions. Their system could find negated expressions both close to and at some distance from the negation cue (signal). The system obtained a precision of 98.6% and a recall of 92.6%.

Mutalik et al. (2001) called their system NegFinder and it was developed by analysing over 40 medical documents for negations patterns and transferring that knowledge to the classical tools for compiler constructions, Lex and Yacc. By using this technique they were able match the negations by complete phrase matching for controlling the negation scope: they used prepositions and conjunctions as well as personal and relative pronouns. NegFinder achieved a precision of 91.8% and a recall of 95.7%.

Rokach et al. (2008) used clinical narratives reports manually annotated for negation a total of 1766 negated instances. Several machine learning algorithms were compared: HMM, CRF, decision trees and AdaBoost, Cascade DTs with longest common subsequence (LCS). Cascade DTs with LCS gave the best results with a precision of 94.4%, a recall of 97.4% and F-score of 95.9%.

7.5.3 *Factuality Detection*

As mentioned in Sect. 4.6.2, clinical text contains a lot of speculative expressions. These expressions are in a range from completely affirmed through different levels of speculation to completely non-affirmed. It is of great importance to distinguish these expressions. First to detect them and then to grade them. There have been several studies, some initial approaches were mentioned in Sect. 7.5.2, along with pure negation detection.

Szarvas (2008) describes a trial to automatically identify speculative sentences in radiology reports, he used the annotated Bioscope corpus in his approach. The machine learning package Maxent based on the maximum entropy framework gave an F-score of 0.64 and F-scores up to 0.821, when using both advanced feature selection mechanisms and external dictionaries as support.

Morante and Daelemans (2009) obtained a precision of up to 100%, and a recall of 97.5% and an F-score of 0.988 on negation signal, using Tilburg Memory Based Learner (TiMBL) together with a list of manually constructed cue words for training and detecting the negations and speculations. To detect the negation scope, they used

- Program modules for detection of
  - Symptom and diagnosis
  - Negation
  - Uncertainty
  - Period of time

- 76-year old woman with hypertension and angina pectoris. Possible heart attack 2 years ago. Admitted to hospital with central chest pain without radiation.

Fig. 7.5 Program modules for clinical named entity recognition (NER) applied on a clinical text. Symptom and diagnosis are sometimes interchangeable. *Possible* weakens factuality, negation remove the factuality of the symptom or diagnosis. Finally, the temporal modifier *2 years ago* takes the occurrence of the diagnosis back in time

three different machine learning systems: SVM, CRF++ and TiMBL, which gave F-scores of 0.893, 0.863 and 0.804 respectively.[17]

Velupillai (2011) defined six different levels, namely *Certainly Positive, Probably Positive, Possibly Positive, Possibly Negative, Probably Negative* and *Certainly Negative*, see Sect. 4.6.2 for details. Velupillai obtained an F-score of 0.699 using all classes, and an F-score of 0.762 using merged classes, with the CRF++ classifier.

Velupillai et al. (2014) carried out and described the porting of the English pyConTextNLP to Swedish pyConTextSwe. pyConTextSwe is dictionary based and can distinguish between four assertion classes (*definite existence, probable existence, probable negated existence* and *definite negated existence*) and two binary classes (*existence yes/no* and *uncertainty yes/no*). pyConTextSwe obtained the following evaluation: F-score 0.81 (overall) and for each of the assertion classes F-scores of 0.88 (definite existence), 0.81 (probable existence), 0.55 (probable negated existence) and 0.63 (definite negated existence). For the two binary classes (existence yes/no) and (uncertainty yes/no), the F-scores were 0.97/0.87 and 0.78/0.86 respectively.

The French version of NegEx (Grouin et al. 2011) mentioned in Sect. 7.5.2 can also process possible negations.

Figure 7.5 demonstrates how these modules will operate on a clinical text. Other clinical entities that can be recognised are drug names, drug doses and body parts.

7.5.4 Relative Processing (Family History)

Findings and disorders mentioned in the patient record may concern relatives of the patient for heredity reasons. Physicians diagnosing a patient search for different

[17]The measurement has changed to a dimensionless quantity from the original percentage in Morante and Daelemans (2009), since F-score is measured as a dimensionless quantity.

His father had high hypertension, and now present with a fever of 39° C lasting two days.

or another possible option is:
Hypertension in family (when it is related to the family of the patient).

or finally:
Had hypertension two years ago (which is a temporal relation).

Fig. 7.6 Examples of excerpts from a clinical texts containing relatives or temporal entities

symptoms, when reading the patient record if one symptom was connected to a family member, or family history, or happened long time ago it may not be valid for the current case, see Fig. 7.6 for different examples of these phenomena.

Clinical text mining to identify relatives and distinguish their symptoms from the patient being treated is sometimes called *relative processing* or *experiencer*.[18] Here a finer grained processing can also be carried out and distinguishing the closeness of the relation to the patient: *1st degree relative* or *2nd degree relative* etc. (South et al. 2009). Relative named entity recognition can also be found in the de-identification of patient records where the category *relative* is used. Entities of the relative class are for example *father, mother, son, daughter, brother, grandfather* and *grandmother*.

7.5.5 *Temporal Processing*

One other important task in clinical text mining is to distinguish where in a timeline a symptom, disorder or event is placed or occurred. Is the symptom a current one or a symptom that occurred one week, one month or some years ago?

The reason for having temporal treatment of symptoms is related to the way physicians reason about diseases, which symptoms occurred just before the disorder? But also to understand care progression and remove non-relevant symptoms that should not be included in the diagnosis. This is similar to the case with negated symptoms in the text. The negated symptoms are not relevant for the diagnosis.

In Fig. 7.7 we can see some of the aspects of temporality in a clinical text. For example, it is important to know that *the chest pain with radiation* preceded the *angina pectoris*, so the chest pain with radiation is a symptom of angina pectoris.

In the early 1980s within Artificial Intelligence Allen (1984) carried out research in natural language processing and problem solving that included understanding time aspects. Allen defined seven time relations: *before, meets, overlaps, is-finished-by, contains, starts* and *equals*.

[18]Experiencer trigger lists, https://github.com/chapmanbe/negex/blob/master/genConText/experiencer_triggers.txt. Accessed 2018-01-11.

76-year old woman with hypertension and angina pectoris. Possible heart attack 2 years ago. Admitted to hospital with central chest pain with radiation. Oct 23, underwent PCI,[a] and now present with a fever of 39°C lasting two days. (Note that admission date is October 18, 2012 obtained from an administrative data source).

Fig. 7.7 Fictive clinical text showing the different temporal aspects that have to be treated by a computer program. [a]PCI stands for Percutaneous Coronary Intervention usually meaning inserting a stent into one of the coronary arteries (in the heart) that is too narrow, to open it to prevent angina pectoris or save the patient for myocardial infarction (AMI), commonly known as a heart attack

Several approaches from the 1990s and onward have been used to process temporal relations in clinical text. For a nice overview see Meystre et al. (2008) but also Velupillai et al. (2015), and for state of the art specifically in temporal applications see (Sun et al. 2013b).

Zhou and Hripcsak (2007) made an early overview of different approaches to temporal reasoning in what they call medical natural language processing. The authors distinguish three main approaches:

1. Temporal reasoning based on theories and models from Artificial Intelligence.
2. Frameworks based on needs from clinical applications.
3. Resolving issues around temporal granularity and uncertainty.

Zhou and Hripcsak (2007) also discuss how to process absolute and relative time and how to combine structured time points with time points mentioned in unstructured free text.

Jung et al. (2011) have a nice example on building timelines from clinical narrative using a deep semantic natural language understanding, and building and visualising the result.

In Sun et al. (2013b) the authors give examples of typical questions that can be raised in a clinical context, such as:

- What medication was the patient on before the surgery?
- How often did the patient experience headache before the treatment?
- What symptoms did the patient experience after taking Aspirin for 3 days?

In Zhou et al. (2005) there is an approach using MedLEE adapted for temporal tagging of clinical narratives. The authors did not use any standard but they invented the whole temporal processing framework.

Identifying temporal relations needs two basic cornerstones to stand on, first the identification of clinical entities such as findings, disorders and the temporal expressions date, time and duration and secondly determining the order these occurred.

A recent book analysing temporal ordering for events and time points is the book by Derczynski (2017).

TimeML and TIMEX3

One method to annotate temporal expressions is to use the *TIMEX* format from the named entity research area (Chinchor and Robinson 1997), which basically is date and time expressions. TIMEX was developed in the *TIMEX3* version and used in the *markup language for temporal and event expressions (TimeML)*, the TimeML language is described in Pustejovsky et al. (2003).

TimeML is a specification language for temporal expressions in natural language and follows the ISO 8601 standard. TimeML treats four problems in event and temporal expression markup according to Pustejovsky et al. (2003):

- Time stamping of events (identifying an event and anchoring it in time).
- Ordering events with respect to one another (lexical versus discourse properties of ordering).
- Reasoning with contextually underspecified temporal expressions (temporal functions such as *last week* and *two weeks before*).
- Reasoning about the persistence of events (how long does an event or the outcome of an event last).

HeidelTime

Strötgen and Gertz (2010) developed the rule-based system temporal tagger *HeidelTime* (from Heidelberg University, Germany) that extracts temporal expressions from text into the TIMEX3 format, which is part of the TimeML standard. The HeidelTime system is modular and therefore easy to adapt to other languages. HeidelTime is currently available for 13 languages: English, German, Dutch, Vietnamese, Arabic, Spanish, Italian, French, Chinese, Russian, Croatian, Estonian and Portuguese.

i2b2 Temporal Relations Challenge

The Sixth Informatics for the Informatics for Integrating Biology and the Bedside (i2b2), Natural Language Processing Challenge for Clinical Records focused on the temporal relations in clinical narratives: 310 discharge summaries were annotated for temporal information. 18 teams participated in the challenge.

HeidelTime was adapted to English clinical text tagging in the i2b2 challenge and obtained the best results of all systems (Sun et al. 2013a).

In these challenges, annotated data is usually released for the different teams to train and develop on, then *held out test data* (data not used for training or developing) is given to the participating team to evaluate their results.

In the i2b2 temporal relations challenge there were three concepts to identify: the TIMEX3 temporal expressions such as TIMES, DATES and DURATION. FREQUENCY (also called SET), and EVENTs denoting an event or action and TLINKs corresponding to a temporal relation denoting the order (e.g. before, after, simultaneous, overlapping, etc.) of an EVENT and a TIMEX3, or two EVENTs or two TIMEX3s.

This follows exactly Styler et al. (2014) who claim that there are three types of temporal relations:

- Relations between two events.
- Relations between two times.
- Relations between a time and an event.

Some TIMEX3s are the frequency of an event, as for example *twice daily* as in *Claritin* 30 mg *twice daily* or *once a week at bedtime*.

Styler et al. (2014) present their approach where they used the Thyme corpus and extracted 1254 de-identified notes written in English from a large healthcare practice (the Mayo Clinic).

Two independent annotators annotated the clinical notes for the entities, EVENT, TIMEX3 and LINK. In total 15,769 EVENTS, 1429 TIMEX3s and 7927 LINKs were found. Inter-annotator agreement as resolved by F-score was 0.80 for EVENT and TIMEX but 0.50 for LINK.

The authors applied the ClearTK-TimeML system which is based on the SVM machine learning algorithm and trained for the Clinical TempEval 2013 competition, on their annotated Thyme corpus and obtained F-scores of 0.496 for TIMEX3, 0.366 for EVENT and 0.204 for LINK. The low performance can be explained by the difference in domains.

Styler et al. (2014) also discuss a new type of TIMEX3 expressions, called PREPOSTEXP, covering a span of text before or after an EVENT (operation). These temporal expressions are *preoperative, postoperative* and *intraoperative*, meaning before, after an operation and between operations. In Styler et al. (2014) the Thyme corpus is also described. Thyme is an acronym for *Temporal Histories of Your Medical Events* and the corpus contains 1254 de-identified notes, within the brain cancer and colon cancer domains. The colon cancer notes contain both clinical notes and pathology reports. The corpus and the guidelines for the temporal annotations can be found online.[19]

[19]Thyme corpus, http://thyme.healthnlp.org. Accessed 2018-01-11.

Temporal Processing for Swedish Clinical Text

For Swedish, Velupillai (2014) carried out a rule-based approach where she adapted the rule-based system temporal tagger HeidelTime to Swedish and applied it to a small subset of Swedish intensive care unit patient records. The adapted version of HeidelTime obtained a precision of 92% and recall of 66%.

Temporal Processing for French Clinical Text

Hamon and Grabar (2014) adapted the rule-based system temporal tagger HeidelTime to French as well as to English. The adaptation consisted of adding more rules to HeidelTime to deal with complicated clinical text (164 rules in English and 47 rules in French).

Both the French and English adapted version, of HeidelTime performed better in processing clinical text than the general purpose version processing general text. For French the performance increased from an F-score of 0.918 to an F-score of 0.942 for general text and medical text respectively. For English the performance increased more, from an F-score of 0.655 to an F-score of 0.843 for general text and medical text respectively.

Temporal Processing for Portuguese Clinical Text

One piece of research work on Brazilian Portuguese clinical text was carried out by Tissot (2016) in his PhD-thesis. Tissot specifically studied how to detect imprecise temporal expression, for example:

The patient says that he had pneumonia more than 2 years ago. More than 3 months ago. A few days ago. A long time ago. The coming months. When exactly is that?

A very imprecise temporal expression is: *The patient says he had weight loss.* When did the weight loss happen?

The Portuguese clinical corpus used for this study is called the InfoSaude corpus and contains 3360 patient records from general medicine, gynecology, nutrition and psychiatry. It was extracted from the InfoSaude system of the Public Health Department in Florianopolis, Brazil. Tissot also used the English TempEval corpus.

Two systems were developed to identify time expressions, one rule-based called HINX, which was developed using GATE by adapting the standard NLP processing modules to the clinical domain, and one machine learning-based using the SVM algorithm as implemented on LibSVM. Three steps were carried out:

1. Text pre-processing;
2. TIMEX identification; and
3. TIMEX normalisation.

where step 1, is standard in NLP, and step 3, was to determine on the scope of specific imprecise temporal expressions.

Normalisation of imprecise temporal expressions was carried out by interviewing people about how they understand and interpret imprecise temporal expressions and how to normalise them. One approach used was to utilise a fuzzy membership function. The membership function would place an imprecise TIMEX in the timeline to perform the normalisation, for example *3* in the expression *about 3 months* is converted to *90 days*. Part of the normalisation process was to correct spelling errors. The process of building the spelling error detection and correction system was based on both string similarity and a phonetic similarity functionality for Portuguese clinical text.

The HINX system found 503,005 TIMEXs and 52,830 imprecise TIMEXs in the Portuguese InfoSaude corpus among the 3360 patient records; however, the quality of these results was never evaluated since the InfoSaude corpus was not manually annotated.

One finding was that clinical text contained more imprecise temporal expressions, up to 35%, than standard news text or historical text, comprising up to 13%, of the total temporal expressions. The high numbers were found in a British clinical corpus called the SLaM (BRC Case Register) corpus.

7.5.6 *Relation Extraction*

Relation extraction is a classification problem, is this relation holding between these two entities? First the two entities that will hold a relation need to be identified using named (clinical) entity recognition, then the relation has to be established. NER is a well-established research area with F-scores of 0.90 and above, while relation extraction is more difficult and reaches only an F-score around 0.70 (Uzuner et al. 2011). See Sect. 7.5.1 for more on clinical named entity recognition.

Relation extraction is a common task in biomedical text mining when a relation must be established between two molecules, or two chemical substances. Are these two components reacting with each other? A nice overview of different approaches of relation extractions in the biomedical domain can be found in Luo et al. (2016).

In clinical text mining one task is to detect an adverse drug event, by detecting the relation between a drug and a finding or symptom. Is there an indication for this drug and this finding or symptom?

2010 i2b2/VA Challenge Relation Classification Task

Uzuner et al. (2011) have a nice review article on various approaches for detection of clinical relations; however, in their article they have not really defined what is an assertion or a concept or the difference between them. A relation holds between two assertions or two concepts or between a concept and an assertion. A concept or assertion seems to be a medical problem, a test, or a treatment.

The best performing system of ten different systems was by de Bruijn et al. (2011), which obtained both best assertion detection with an F-score of 0.936 and best concept extraction with an F-score of 0.852. These are pre-requisites for relation assertion, which they also obtained the second best results with an F-score of 0.731. The assertion classifier and the relation classifier of de Bruijn et al. used an approach called semi-supervised learning through clustering. The Brown clustering algorithm was used on the unlabelled clinical corpora for the unsupervised approach, and applied the features produced for their supervised approach using a semi-Markov model (de Bruijn et al. 2011).

SVM gave the best results for the relation extraction task for clinical text in the 2010 i2b2/VA challenge (Uzuner et al. 2011).

Other Approaches for Relation Extraction

In a study by Henriksson et al. (2015) a Swedish clinical text containing adverse drug events (ADEs) was annotated for named clinical entities as well as ADE relations. For the named entity annotations *finding, disorder, drug, body part* and *ADE cue* the IAA F-scores were around 0.84. For the semantic relation annotations *indication, adverse drug event, ADE outcome* and *ADE cause* the IAA were lower at around 0.65. For the training and detection of the named entities CRF++ was used together with features extracted from an unsupervised distributional semantics approach, specifically Word2Vec (skip-gram model); for detecting named clinical entities the F-score results were around 0.80, while for relation extraction were much lower around 0.45.

In the study by Bejan and Denny (2014) the authors used 6864 discharge summaries that were annotated by two annotators, finding 958 treatment relations and 9628 non-treatment relations. Two different pre-annotation tools were used, first a tool called SemRep and second their own tool known as the MEDI algorithm, which both extract relations but in different ways. MEDI is a UMLS based pre-annotation tool. 25% of the data was double annotated obtaining an F-score for IAA of 0.979 with a Cohen's kappa of 0.86. For the training the authors used LIBSVM and with 5-fold cross validation obtained an F-score of 0.85.

Bejan and Denny (2014) refer to Roberts et al. (2008) as one of the first attempts to extract relations from clinical text. Roberts et al. (2008) annotated 77 oncology narratives with seven categories of relations, obtaining low IAA with an F-score of 0.47. SVM was used for the training and an F-score of 0.72 was obtained over a class of seven relation types.

7.5.7 Anaphora Resolution

Anaphora resolution sometimes also called *co-reference resolution* is the task of resolving which entity in a sentence, a pronoun or a noun phrase refers to.

The *anaphor* is the pointing back reference (the pronoun or the noun phrase). The *antecedent* is the entity that is referred to by the anaphor. These are also called *markables* or *markable*, which are terms used in the anaphora research area.

The task of determining the antecedent of an anaphor is called anaphora resolution or co-reference resolution. For an example of anaphora see Fig. 7.8.

Some anaphora occur within a sentence, and are called intrasentential anaphors and some anaphora are referring over sentence borders and are called intersentential anaphors.

The anaphora resolution usually takes place by gender and number agreement, but there are also many other ways to resolve the anaphora. Sometimes it is not resolved. The research area of anaphora resolution is well studied in computational linguistics though not completely solved, for a nice overview of the state of the art see (Mitkov 2014).

He (2007) wrote a master's thesis in the area of coreference resolution in discharge summaries using 47 hospital discharge summaries written in English, containing in total 4978 lines of text.

The author let two computer science students annotate the corpus with coreference chains and time stamps. The coreference chains contained five different annotation classes depending whether the coreference was about a person, symptom, disease, medication or test. A *coreference chain* is a line between the antecedent and the following possible anaphors referring to the antecedent in an anaphora resolution system.

The inter-annotator agreement measured by Kappa-value averaged 0.836 over all annotation classes, which is considerably high and corresponds to an easy annotation task.

The training set created was comparably small, in total 649 coreferent pairs, and therefore a lot of features were needed to compensate for the scarce training data.

The time stamp was annotated to distinguish whether a symptom occurred a long time ago or not and was used as a feature. In addition to the time stamps the author also used a set of carefully selected features.

> *76-year old woman with hypertension and angina pectoris. Possible heart attack 2 years ago. Admitted to hospital with central chest pain without radiation. She mentioned her daughter had similar symptoms. She was treated and is fine now.*

Fig. 7.8 Fictive clinical text with a pronominal anaphora, *76-year old woman* is the antecedent and *She* is the anaphor. The pronominal anaphora is not resolved, who is the last *she* in the text referring to? The daughter or the patient? Probably the daughter and not the patient

The machine learning algorithm used for training was the supervised C4.5 Decision Tree algorithm and the author obtained a lowest overall B-CUBED precision of 0.983 and a lowest overall B-CUBED recall of 0.947. B-CUBED precision and recall are specific evaluation metrics constructed for evaluating coreference chains as explained in Bagga and Baldwin (1998).

i2b2 Challenge in Coreference Resolution for Electronic Medical Records

A review on different approaches to resolve the anaphoras in electronic medical records is described in Uzuner et al. (2012). This was part of the Fifth i2b2/VA Workshop on Natural Language Processing Challenges for Clinical Records. In total 20 teams from 29 organisations and from nine different countries participated.

The data used in the challenge comprised progress notes, discharge records, radiology reports and surgical pathology reports from Beth Israel Deaconess Medical Center, Partners Healthcare and University of Pittsburgh Medical Center (UPMC), as well as clinical reports and pathology reports from the Mayo Clinic. All written in English and de-identified, in total there were 978 files.

The data was annotated by two independent annotators for coreference pairs, almost 5646 coreference chains were annotated.

The results from the challenge showed that both the machine learning and the rule-based approaches worked best when augmented with external knowledge. 77.75% of the ground truth chains were correctly predicted by all systems and 95.07% of by at least one system.

7.6 Summary of Basic Building Blocks for Clinical Text Processing

This chapter presented all the steps necessary for performing natural language processing on clinical text, starting with word segmentation and continuing with tokenisation and morphological processing, which encompasses, compound splitting, stemming, abbreviation detection, spell checking and correction, part-of-speech tagging followed by a discussion of syntactical parsing and semantic analysis, such as named entity recognition, different negation detection systems, relation extraction, temporal processing and anaphora resolution.

Usually one or more of these steps need to be carried out but not all of them, since usually only some information needs to be extracted from the text for a specific task. For continued reading see the following books on NLP Mitkov (2005), Jurafsky and Martin (2014) and Clark et al. (2013).

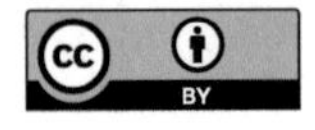

Chapter 8
Computational Methods for Text Analysis and Text Classification

In this chapter the differences between rule-based systems and machine learning-based systems along with their respective pros and cons will be explained. The principles of machine learning-based systems such as Conditional Random Fields (CRF), Support Vector Machines (SVM) and the Weka toolkit supporting several machine learning algorithms and evaluation packages will be presented. For machine learning feature extraction for improving the machine learning results will be described, feature extraction such as POS-tagging, stemming and lemmatisation, as well as statistical calculations based on tf–idf to filter out relevant words. Active learning is used for selecting the optimal data to be annotated. Different machine learning approaches such as topic modelling, distributional semantics and clustering will be presented. Text is preprocessed into different knowledge representations such as vector space model and word space model etc. These representations are adapted for different computational methods. The results produced from both rule-based and machine learning-based systems will be explained. Ready computational linguistic modules for English clinical text mining, such as MedLEE and cTakes will also be presented, as well as some basic tools such as NLTK and GATE, which need to be adapted to clinical text mining.

8.1 Rule-Based Methods

The rule-based method is the classical programming paradigm. A human programmer or software engineer writes rules to mimic the required behavior of a program. The programmer studies a flow chart of how the program should react depending on the, input data to the program. The programmer may also study the input data and the required output data and try to implement this in the program. The rules can be any type of format, a grammar for parsing text, regular expressions to extract parts of

H. Dalianis, *Clinical Text Mining*, https://doi.org/10.1007/978-3-319-78503-5_8

```
grep -o -P -e "(\d{6}|\d{8}) (-|)\d{4}(\W|$)" personnummer.txt
```

Fig. 8.1 An example of a *regular expression* that would find a Swedish personal identity number, *\d* matches digits, six or eight in a row with a hyphen or not *(-|)* and finally a group of four digits. At the end of the regular expression there is a check for a non-word character *W* and end of the line *$*. The grep command in the Bash shell script of the Linux operating system print lines matching a regular expression applied to a file called "personnummer.txt". This regular expression can be more elaborate by adding features for the century e.g. 1900 and 2000, as well as for 12 months and 31 days, and also checksum for the last four digits

strings, or a number of regular expressions to perform stemming or lemmatisation of words. Rule-based methods are time consuming and require hands-on programming and understanding of the problem to be solved. Rule-based methods are perfect for handling specific problems, but not for processing unexpected input data. See also Sect. 7.4.2 on writing grammars to parse input text and produce output data from a syntax tree. Usually rule-based method obtains high precision and lower recall.

8.1.1 Regular Expressions

Included in rule-based methods are the *regular expressions* also called *regex* or *regexp*.[1] Regexp are very powerful search and string matching techniques to make an exact match on text, words, characters, numerical expressions, non-alphanumeric expressions and parts of them. Regular expressions are available in the Linux operating systems as well as in most programming languages. Regexp are usually used to find, and sometimes replace parts or whole expressions in a text.

An example of using RegExp to find the format of a Swedish personal identity number that contains a six-digit birth date part and four control digits: YYMMDD-NNNN, follows here. A personal identity number is sometimes written in full with four year digits: YYYYMMDD-NNNN, but it can also be the case that it is written without a hyphen: YYMMDDNNNN. Examples of personal identity numbers are *690401-9304, 19690401-9304* or *196904019304*. Therefore, to find all Swedish personal identity numbers in a file called "personnummer.txt" you have to type the following command in Bash shell script of the Linux operating system. Grep in the shell script print lines matching regular expression pattern, see Fig. 8.1.

Of course this can be elaborated, allowing only a maximum 12 months and 31 days, the last four digits are control numbers and these can be also checked.

Regular expressions can be used to find and replace personal identity numbers, telephone numbers and email addresses that are regular and easy to identify for example for de-identification purposes, see Sect. 9.4.

[1] Regular expressions, https://en.wikipedia.org/wiki/Regular_expression. Accessed 2018-01-11.

8.2 Machine Learning-Based Methods

Machine learning is a set of methods that uses previous patterns of behaviour and can generalise a set of rules or behavior from this. Machine learning methods learn from previous patterns. Within machine learning methods we can distinguish between unsupervised methods and supervised methods.

Unsupervised methods utilise training data that is not annotated or preprocessed manually by any human. These unsupervised methods can be different clustering methods, distributional semantics as random indexing or Hidden Markov Models.

Supervised methods use training data that is manually annotated with labels, consequently it is very expensive in terms of human effort and time to produce annotated data for supervised methods. Hence, some supervised methods will first be described, such as Conditional Random Field (CRF) and Support Vector Machine (SVM), and then some unsupervised methods to find semantic relations, such as Latent Semantic Analysis (LSA), Latent Semantic Indexing and Random Indexing as well as text clustering.

Conditional Random Field (CRF) is an efficient machine learning algorithm for detecting named entities in a sequence of data. CRF is related to Hidden Markov Models (HMM) and is a supervised algorithm that needs annotated data. CRF can predict sequences of labels after training. For a thorough description on CRF see Lafferty et al. (2001). There are several implementations of CRF such as CRF++, Stanford NER, and CRF Mallet, to mention some. Stanford NER is a well performing system with an elaborate graphical interface, see Fig. 8.2.

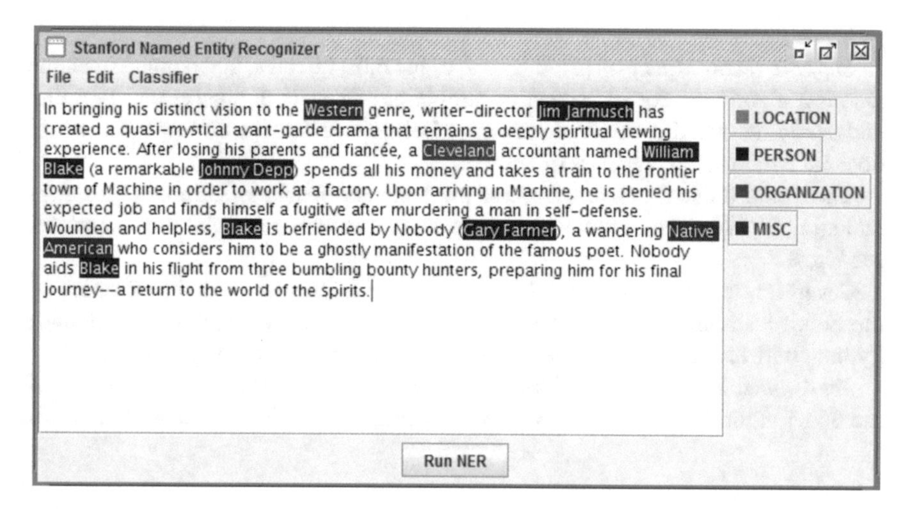

Fig. 8.2 The interface of Stanford NER[a] implementing CRF. [a]Stanford NER, http://www.linguisticsweb.org/doku.php?id=linguisticsweb:tutorials:linguistics_tutorials:automaticannotation:stanford_ner. Accessed 2018-01-11

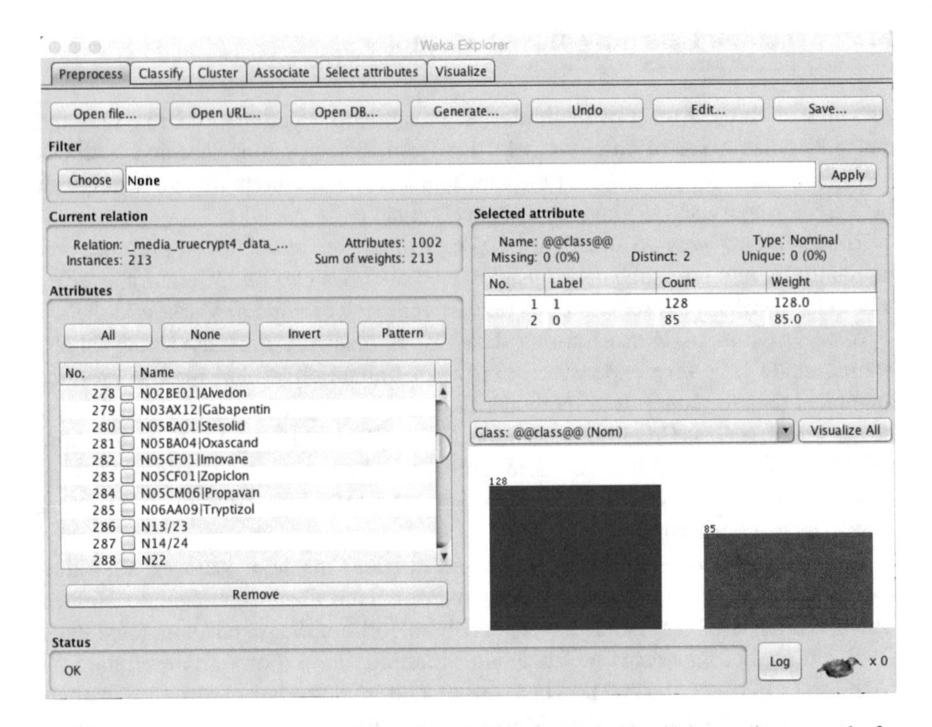

Fig. 8.3 The interface of the Weka toolkit. In this example classifying patient records for healthcare associated infections taken from Ehrentraut et al. (2014). Reprinted with the permission of the authors in Ehrentraut et al. (2014)

Support Vector Machines (SVM) is one of the most effective and popular machine learning algorithms for classification problems. SVM is a supervised algorithm and needs annotated data. SVM can, after training, decide if a concept or a whole document belongs to one class or another.

The Weka toolkit[2] contains several implemented machine learning algorithms including SVM as well as evaluation packages and an elaborated graphical interface, see Fig. 8.3.

Several researchers use the R programming language[3] with its libraries or the Scikit-learn environment[4] which is also based on the programming language Python, both are suitable for performing machine learning-based approaches.

Yet Another Multipurpose CHunk Annotator (YamCha)[5] is an implementation of the SVM algorithm and uses the CoNLL format (which is a standard format for

---

[2]Weka toolkit, http://www.cs.waikato.ac.nz/ml/weka/. Accessed 2018-01-11.

[3]R Project, https://www.r-project.org. Accessed 2018-01-11.

[4]Scikit-learn, http://scikit-learn.org. Accessed 2018-01-11.

[5]YamCha, http://chasen.org/~taku/software/yamcha/. Accessed 2018-01-11.

NLP training and testing) and is therefore suitable to combine with experiments using CRF++ that also use the CoNLL format.

Machine learning-based methods do not need so much programming effort but time to prepare the data in the right format, in other words, to find the optimal knowledge representation and the most efficient features in the data to be used. Supervised methods require time consuming manual annotation of the data to be used for training (and evaluation).

Machine learning-based methods generally obtain high recall and lower precision. For more details on machine learning see Alpaydin (2014).

8.2.1 Features and Feature Selection

Features represent certain aspects of the training data and are used as input to the machine learning tools. Features are usually produced by different preprocessing tools such as taggers.

Each word's POS-tag such as *determiner, subject, predicate, adjective, adverb, preposition etc.* may be used as a feature, but also features such as if the word contain an initial capital letter, the length of the word, if it is numerical token, the surrounding word's features, etc., for more details see Dalianis and Boström (2012).

Stemmers produce stems and lemmatisers lemmas that may be used as features, for more details see Dalianis and Boström (2012).

Dictionary matching means to select the words and arbitrary features of tokens that have a match with some known dictionary, such as ICD-10, SNOMED-CT, MeSH etc., for more details see Skeppstedt et al. (2014).

Statistical calculations such as the term frequency–inverse document frequency (*tf–idf*) of tokens in the document collection may be used as features, for more details see Ehrentraut et al. (2014).

Stop word filtering means to remove the most common (non-significant) words from the document collections, which account around 40% of all tokens.

Other methods to produce features is to use distributional semantics applied on large unsupervised corpora to extract features from the corpora and apply the features on a smaller subset of annotated text, for more details see Henriksson et al. (2014).

The Weka toolkit has both a built-in feature extraction mechanism as well as feature selection and feature optimisation algorithms.

Term Frequency–Inverse Document Frequency, tf–idf

To find the statistically most significant word in a document collection there is a statistical calculation called *term frequency–inverse document frequency, tf–idf*, it comprises of two separate calculations: term frequency (tf) of a word in a particular document multiplied with the inverse document frequency (idf) of the same word over the document collection. The product gives the tf–idf weight of a specific word meaning the significance of this word within a particular document. Here follows the definitions of the used terms to calculate tf–idf:

- The *term frequency (tf)* corresponds to the number of times a word occurs in a particular document.
- The *document frequency (df)* corresponds to the number of documents that contains a specific word at least once.
- The *number of documents (N)* corresponds to the number of documents in a document collection.
- The *inverse document frequency (idf)* of a word calculates how unique or common a word is across a document collection. A unique word has a high idf, while a common term has a low idf. Idf for a specific word is calculated by dividing the number of documents *(N)* with the document frequency *(df)* for a specific word in the document collection. The logarithmic function is applied on the result to scale the quote for the length of the documents. Hence, normalising the result and avoiding that words in long documents will obtain high idf. Words in long documents tend to be repeated and consequently obtain high term frequency. For the formula on idf see (8.1) and for the formula on tf–idf see (8.2).

$$idf = log\left(\frac{N}{df}\right) \tag{8.1}$$

$$tf\text{–}idf = tf \times idf \tag{8.2}$$

Words with a high tf–idf weight are more significant than words with a lower tf–idf weight. For further details regarding tf–idf see Van Rijsbergen (1979) and Manning et al. (2008).

One preprocessing method is therefore to filter out words with a high tf–idf weight that are words with high significance, to be used as training data in a machine learning algorithm, while words with a low tf–idf weight usually coincide with stop words, meaning words with low significance.

Vector Space Model

Another similarity measurement between documents apart of tf–idf is the *vector space model* that considers each word in a document to be a vector. All the word vectors summarised gives a measurement for the document. Comparing two documents in the vector space model is carried out by comparing the angle between the two document vectors, if there is a small angle between the two vectors, the corresponding documents are considered to be closely related. The vector space model is used in information retrieval where one of the vectors is the query vector.

The vector space model can be used both for measuring the similarity between two documents, where the document vector consists of the sum of all word vectors and also for measuring the similarity of two words by comparing the corresponding word vectors.

Cosine similarity is a measurement sprung from the vector space model, indicating the closeness of two vectors by calculating the dot product between them. If the number is 1 or close to 1 then the cosine similarity also shows similarity between the document vectors. If words are compared for similarity, then the word vectors are compared, or more precisely the angle between the word vectors, the smaller angle between the word vectors the more similar words.

8.2.2 Active Learning

Various *active learning* methods for machine learning have been developed. The aim of active learning is to reduce the amount of manual annotation effort needed to obtain training data. Active learning helps to select the most information dense and variated training data to be annotated which contributes to the best and optimal training examples. The process of active learning is often iterative. Optimal data is data not seen or used by the algorithm previously. This optimal data can be selected by a machine or by a human (Settles 2009).

Olsson (2009) has also written a nice overview of active learning within natural language processing. In his PhD thesis Olsson (2008) proposes his method BootMark that includes three steps:

(a) Manual annotation of a set of documents;
(b) Bootstrapping—active machine learning for the purpose of selecting which document to annotate next; and
(c) Mark up of the remaining unannotated documents of the original corpus using pre-tagging with revision.

The BootMark method is proved to require fewer manually annotated documents for the training of a named entity recogniser, and is better than training on randomly selected documents.

Boström and Dalianis (2012) used active learning for a de-identification annotation experiment, and found that both random selection and selecting the most certain examples outperformed the standard active learning strategy of selecting the most uncertain examples. The reason for this can be a skewed class distribution when selecting the most uncertain examples.

Kholghi et al. (2015) used three different active learning algorithms to decide on which unlabeled instances to annotate next. The studied algorithms were: supervised approach (Sup), information density (ID) and least confidence (LC). The LC algorithm gave the best results. The study reports on a range from 77% to 46% of savings for sequences, tokens, and concepts.

8.2.3 Pre-Annotation with Revision or Machine Assisted Annotation

Pre-annotation with revision[6] is related to active learning. A small set of annotated data is used to start the machine learning process. The presented learned data is reviewed and corrected by a human, and the new annotated data is entered again into the machine learning system to improve the system. This is an iterative process (Olsson 2008).

Pre-annotation[7] means to machine-annotate text before the human annotator receives it to support him or her in the manual annotation process. The pre-annotations are manually corrected and missing annotations are added. The pre-annotations may also be corrected by the human annotator if the pre-annotations are wrong. The corrected annotated text is entered into the machine learning system and the performance of the system is hopefully improved.

A study on pre-annotation and revision is presented in Hanauer et al. (2013). The authors use the MITRE Identification Scrubber Toolkit (MIST) for de-identification. They use ten clinical notes for an initial annotation for de-identification and then training the system, then they pre-annotate another ten notes, correct the annotations, train the system, pre-annotate another ten notes, and do that 21 times. At the end they increase the sample with 20 and 40 notes so in total 220 notes were annotated. For each round the annotation time decreased, and the F-score increased to 0.95 from 0.89 with the initial ten notes. In total 8 h annotation time was used for 21 rounds, the initial ten note round took 33 min with the last round just needing 15 min.

Lingren et al. (2014) showed that pre-annotation of clinical trial announcements (documents) made a time saving for annotation in the range of 13.85–21.5% per entity. The annotators annotated 9002 medical named entities, mainly disease/disorder and sign/symptom entities.

Skeppstedt (2013) suggested one approach in pre-annotation inspired by Olsson (2008). Skeppstedt used the CRF system for pre-annotating unlabelled data. Instead of using the standard method of presenting one pre-annotation, the annotator is presented with two possible pre-annotations. The annotator, therefore, always has to make an active choice between two options, which has the potential to reduce bias. The two possible pre-annotations presented are the ones considered as most likely by the trained CRF model. They are, however, presented in a random order, to avoid a bias towards the most likely pre-annotation, see Fig. 8.4. This approach has not

[6] In this book pre-tagging is called pre-annotation.

[7] Pre-annotation is also called machine assisted annotation.

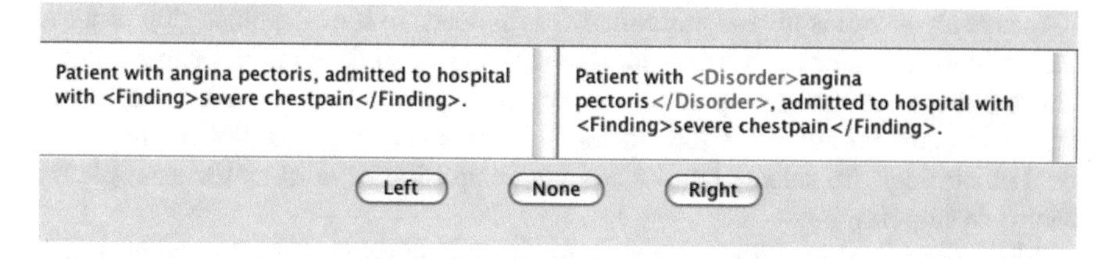
Patient with angina pectoris, admitted to hospital with <Finding>severe chestpain</Finding>.
Patient with <Disorder>angina pectoris</Disorder>, admitted to hospital with <Finding>severe chestpain</Finding>.
Left
None
Right

Fig. 8.4 A simple program for choosing between two alternative annotations, one pre-annotated and one manually annotated. The example is a constructed example in English (Figure taken from Figure 1 in Skeppstedt 2013. © 2013 Reprinted with the permission of ACL and the author. Published in Skeppstedt 2013)

yet been evaluated, but the results from Olsson (2008) indicate that pre-annotation is the right way to go.

One other possibility would be to present the annotator's previous annotation and the one the machine proposes to the annotator, without of course informing them which one is human-made or machine generated, and then the annotator can choose which is the correct one, thereby obtaining the optimal annotation.

Skeppstedt et al. (2017) have developed their method of pre-annotation and active learning in a prototype called PAL, Pre-annotation and Active Learning. Where the annotator only is receiving the most optimal data to annotate for each annotation round. PAL is fully integrated with the BRAT annotation tool and is freely available to download from GitHub.[8]

8.2.4 Clustering

Clustering of documents is in contrast to categorisation (or classification) not predefined. Categorisation means to assign documents in predefined categories according to some manual or rule-based process. Clustering, on the other hand, is a completely unsupervised method for grouping documents, that contain similar meaning bearing words, or are similar in some way in the same cluster. Clustering is an indeterministic process not (always) knowing the number of final clusters and their content beforehand. The process is deterministic in the way that the results will be the same each time the clustering starts. Clustering can also produce overlapping clusters, meaning that a document can be assigned in two or more clusters. Clustering needs a similarity measure between documents, the cosine similarity is often used as a measure but also the tf–idf scheme.

There are two main algorithms for clustering: partitioning and hierarchical algorithms. One well-known partitioning algorithm is the *K-means algorithm*. The

[8]PAL, https://github.com/mariask2/PAL-A-tool-for-Pre-annotation-and-Active-Learning. Accessed 2018-01-11.

K-means algorithm is given k random words as seeds to start the clustering process, then calculate cluster centroids (centre of gravity) try to fit them into nearest initial cluster, check for a stopping condition, regroup clusters, one per cluster centroid, let each document belong to the cluster with the most similar centroid, until some final clusterings are selected and a stopping condition is valid as for example the centroids stop moving.

Since the initial partitions are random the final clustering results are also non-deterministic, using the same data but different random k seed words.

Hierarchical algorithms are on the other hand deterministic and create a clustering hierarchy. The hierarchical algorithms can work top-down or bottom-up. One hierarchical algorithm is the *agglomerative clustering algorithm*, which begins by putting each document in its own cluster. The n clusters that are most similar to each other are then merged into one new cluster and the worst cluster is split into n new clusters, the splitting process repeats until a stopping condition is valid. Usually n is equal to 2. For a nice overview of the area see Rosell (2009).

For an open source search results clustering engine see Carrot^2.[9]

8.2.5 Topic Modelling

Topic modelling is, in contrary to clustering, focused on finding topics in one or more documents and then building a model of topics. Of course longer documents may contain more than one topic. Topic modelling is an unsupervised method. The method assumes that words originate from different topics and are used in a mixed way in a document or corpus. The topic modelling algorithm tries to gather all words that encompass one topic and group them in that topic. The process is iterative and continues until a likely distribution of words is put in each topic. One document or corpus can hence contain several topics. There will of course be more words than topics, since each topic contain several words. Topic modelling and clustering are related in such way that the same topics from different documents can be clustered and hence their corresponding documents. One algorithm often used to perform topic modelling is the Latent Dirichlet Allocation (LDA). For a nice overview of topic modelling see Blei (2012).

8.2.6 Distributional Semantics

The basis of the *distributional hypothesis* is that a word is described by its context. Two words are synonyms or more exactly associonyms if they are used in the same or similar context several times in different documents, which is what creates the

[9] Carrot^2, https://project.carrot2.org. Accessed 2018-01-11.

distributional semantics. The semantics of words are described by their context, or their distribution in the corpus. For each unique word in the corpus a context vector is constructed and a word space model is constructed. A *word space model* is a mathematical model of the corpus that contains information about the distribution of the different words. A distribution describes each word's context in form of other words. This method or the result of the method is also called *word embeddings*.

The first theoretical approach for distributional semantics was latent semantic analysis and it was first implemented in *latent semantic indexing*; however, the method was difficult to scale, so a faster method was later implemented called *Random Indexing (RI)* that reduced the dimensionality for the indexing and hence improved performance, see Sahlgren (2006).

An implementation of random indexing by Martin Duneld, can be found online,[10] another possibility is to use the popular *word2vec* implementation of distributional semantics[11] (Mikolov et al. 2013).

8.2.7 Association Rules

One method to reduce the complexity of big data for text mining (and data mining) is to use association rules, which is a method developed by Agrawal and Srikant (1994). Association rules use statistics to find patterns in large amounts of data and replace the data with rules that generalise or associate. The method was used in clinical text mining by Boytcheva et al. (2017a) for 300,000 outpatient records and 1425 health forum postings, both in Bulgarian. The authors tried through association rules to find attribute-value pairs. An example of an attribute is *cardiovascular system* and a value is for example *rhythmic norm frequent heartrate*.

This method generates a great number of rules by performing post processing, the rules with the highest statistical significance are selected. This method identified relations even when the attribute-value pairs were from apart from each other in the text. First as a preprocessing step the authors performed stemming on the text before generating the association rules. The authors used a ready program package called SPMP[12] for the association rules generation. The result is evaluated with something called Lift value, which is a measure on how well these rules manage to associate; the authors obtained a Lift value on 12.21, which is very good, as a Lift value of over 1.1 is considered good.

[10]JavaSDM: A Java Package for Random Indexing, http://www.csc.kth.se/tcs/humanlang/tools.html. Accessed 2018-01-11.

[11]word2vec, https://code.google.com/p/word2vec/. Accessed 2018-01-11.

[12]SPMP, http://www.philippe-fournier-viger.com/spmf/index.php?link=download.ph. Accessed 2018-01-11.

8.3 Explaining and Understanding the Results Produced

Humans trust results if they are explained and if they can be validated. This was the case with the traditional rule-based expert systems of the 1980s.

Generally, rule-based systems or logic-based systems are comprehensible since they are constructed by humans. The programmer can, for each step, explain to the user why something happened and for what reason, while machine learning systems in contrast analyse several thousands examples mathematically or statistically, and then produces a number of rules or behaviours, which in turn give a result. For example, some specific input data give some specific output data.

Machine learning systems are not very good in general of giving explanations or feedback to the user, however some machine learning algorithms such as decision trees can give some explanation of how they reached a result; linear additive systems can also give some abstract explanation, systems such as Naïve-Bayes, logistic regression and linear Support Vector Machines. These algorithms can demonstrate how the weight for each feature impacted the results (Stumpf et al. 2009).

8.4 Computational Linguistic Modules for Clinical Text Processing

There are two off-the-shelf systems that are mentioned in the research literature, one is the *Medical Language Extraction and Encoding System (MedLEE)*, by Friedman et al. (1995) the other one is *clinical Text Analysis and Knowledge Extraction System (cTAKES)*[13] by Savova et al. (2010). Both systems are ready to use with integrated clinical dictionaries, terminologies and classifications (in English).

cTAKES is an open source NLP toolkit based on UIMA and on the Apache OpenNLP toolkit.[14] It has all the basic NLP processing functionalities for English, such as a tokeniser, a POS-tagger, a named entity recogniser, negation detection, machine learning functionality etc. cTakes is currently used at the Mayo Clinic in Rochester, Minnesota, USA.

MedLEE contains a preprocessor, a rule-based parser, a composer and an encoder. The encoder matches entities in the text with entities in UMLS or SNOMED, or other vocabularies. MedLEE was developed academically but is now a commercial tool. MedLEE is in daily use for clinical decision support at the New York—Presbyterian Hospital (Friedman 2005).

A newer off-the-shelf system is *Clinical Language Annotation, Modelling and Processing Toolkit (CLAMP).*[15] CLAMP is a Java, and Eclipse based annotation

[13]cTakes, https://en.wikipedia.org/wiki/CTAKES. Accessed 2018-01-11.

[14]Apache, OpenNLP , https://en.wikipedia.org/wiki/OpenNLP. Accessed 2018-01-11.

[15]CLAMP, http://clamp.uth.edu. Accessed 2018-01-11.

and NLP toolkit for clinical text. CLAMP has built-in modules for the standard NLP processing steps for English text. CLAMP also has a built-in UMLS encoder.

8.5 NLP Tools: UIMA, GATE, NLTK etc

Here follow a presentation of various ready to use NLP tools. One standard is *Unstructured Information Management Architecture (UIMA)*[16] from IBM for content analytics. It was developed to process unstructured information such as natural language text, speech, images or videos. Another standard that is well-used is *General Architecture for Text Engineering (GATE)*[17] written in Java. GATE was originally developed at the University of Sheffield. Today GATE can process the following languages: English, Chinese, Arabic, Bulgarian, French, German, Hindi, Italian, Cebuano, Romanian, Russian, Danish and Welsh. Another well-known toolkit is the *Natural Language Toolkit (NLTK)*,[18] which was developed in the programming language Python, see Bank and Schierle (2012). Some Java-based NLP tools are:

- LingPipe, http://alias-i.com/lingpipe/
- Stanford CoreNLP, http://stanfordnlp.github.io/CoreNLP/
- OpenNLP Apache, http://opennlp.apache.org/
- Freeling, http://nlp.lsi.upc.edu/freeling/
  (All links accessed 2018-01-11.)

8.6 Summary of Computational Methods for Text Analysis and Text Classification

This chapter presented rule-based methods and continued with machine learning methods such as CRF, SVM and Random Forest, their differences, weaknesses and strengths were compared and explained along with when to use them. For machine learning preprocessing of training data was described, including feature selection. Various knowledge representations of text were presented. Tools as the Stanford NER for CRF and the Weka toolkit supporting a large number of machine learning algorithms were presented. Within machine learning, active learning was discussed, a method for selecting the most optimal data for annotation, continuing with pre-tagging with revision, a method for improving the manual annotation work, with respect to time and quality. Clustering, topic modelling and distributional semantics

[16]UIMA Wikipedia, https://en.wikipedia.org/wiki/UIMA. Accessed 2018-01-11.

[17]GATE, https://gate.ac.uk. Accessed 2018-01-11.

[18]NLTK 3.0 documentation, http://www.nltk.org. Accessed 2018-01-11.

were also explained. Machine learnings algorithms that can explain their results were presented. Various open tools for clinical text mining such as cTakes, NLTK, GATE and Stanford Core NLP were mentioned.

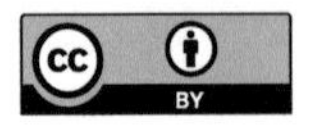

Chapter 9
Ethics and Privacy of Patient Records for Clinical Text Mining Research

There is an abundance of electronic patient records produced today within healthcare. These records contain valuable information on symptoms and disorders, reasoning to determine on the diagnosis and the treatment of the patient, but also on adverse events the patient might have experienced. The whole process of obtaining access to electronic patient records for research is complicated and requires certain steps. This chapter will describe the process of applying for of an ethical permission, data extraction and safe storage of sensitive data. Sensitive data in that sense it is personal data that can identify individuals. Clinical free text extraction require often to identify the sensitive data, so-called de-identification, followed by replacing the identified sensitive data with fake data, so-called pseudonymisation. Privacy preserving methods will also be discussed when connecting the data to other sources and databases there is a risk of re-identification and to avoid this privacy preserving data linkage has to be carried out.

9.1 Ethical Permission

In Sweden and in many other countries ethical permission is needed to perform research on health related data that involves humans. Therefore, first of all an *ethical permission* is needed from an *ethical review board* before any research involving patient records can be carried out. The ethical review board is used by medical researchers applying for permission to perform research involving humans or animals. In the case of clinical text mining, no experiments on humans or animals are carried out but a large amount of data is studied. Data in the form of patient records that contain information about people who have not been asked if they want to participate in any experiment. Usually each individual is asked to agree to participate in a research project, however, in our case we are studying information that is de-identified and no individual can be singled out. The data is also on an

H. Dalianis, *Clinical Text Mining*, https://doi.org/10.1007/978-3-319-78503-5_9

aggregated level and not at an individual level, hence we do not study specific people.

The planned research has to be described in an *application for ethical review* (in Swedish: Etikprövningsansökan) by the researcher, which is addressed to the ethical review board. In the ethical review application, the experiments, the possible outcome and also how the data will be stored are described. The research shall of course not harm any individual and aims to be a benefit for healthcare and humanity. The review board then decides if the research is approved and can be carried out.

As previously mentioned the law in Sweden says that consent must be given by the patient before his or her data can be used for research; however, the patient records used in this research are de-identified meaning that the patient's identity is unknown. According to the Swedish Personal Data Act, (in Swedish) Personuppgiftslagen (1998:204), also abbreviated to PUL, personal information is all type of information that can be linked to a physical person, if it cannot be linked then it is not personal information.

However, in the free text of the patient records there is sometimes mentioned information that may identify the patient, as for example telephone numbers of relatives, (for example the *patient's wife Mary's phone number is 081-590 29 38*), in these cases the patient can be considered to be identifiable and hence the patient has to either be asked for consent to be part of the research project, or the identifiable parts removed.

A overview of the process of obtaining clinical data Internationally, in Australia and in Finland is described in Suominen (2012) in Australia, Austria, Finnish, Swiss and the USA is described in Suominen et al. (2017).

9.2 Social Security Number

After the review board has approved the application for ethical review the research can be carried out. The hospital is contacted (again) with the approval from the ethical review board and then the hospital management decides if the hospital can hand out data for research. This decision can also be taken at a clinical unit level for each clinical unit, but it is better to have the hospital management as the decision maker, since the research project can get access to more data from *all* clinical units. In some cases extra sensitive data for patients treated for psychiatric reasons or sexually transmitted diseases has to be left out of the study.

Before obtaining the data from the hospital the personal names and the social security numbers must be removed. The social security number is replaced by a serial number. At the hospital a key is generated and stored to link the serial number to the social security number so the patient can be tracked later, or the data linked to another register.

Observe also the Scandinavian countries, have a unique personal identity number (in Swedish: *personnummer*) used for all contact with the authorities. (each Scandinavian country has its own system of personal identity numbers).

In Sweden a personal identity number is given to each individual at birth and is kept for the whole life span. Immigrants are given a number on arrival to the country, a number which is also kept for their whole life. The advantage of this number is that a person or a patient can be followed when admitted to the hospital but also when discharged from or re-admitted to the hospital. The same number is also used in other registries, such as the prescribed drugs registry, the cause of death registry, or a cancer registry and business registries. However, to connect different registries permission is needed from different authorities. When linking registries, a serial number is used instead of the personal identity number to make the transaction anonymous.

After obtaining ethical permission for the research, the researcher needs to get access to the anonymised patient records to perform the research. The access to the patient records may be cumbersome technically if there is no easy way to extract the data from the electronic patient record system. However, if the data is extracted it is necessary to store it at a safe place at the research unit or at the hospital. A safe place that cannot be accessed by any unauthorised personnel.

9.3 Safe Storage

If the data is stored at the academic institution and not at the hospital certain steps have to be carried out. In the case of Stockholm University with HEALTH BANK the following applies (Dalianis et al. 2015): The de-identified patient records for research are stored on a server that is encrypted and password protected, without any Internet connection. The server is locked to the server rack. The server rack is in a server room in that in turn is locked and alarmed, and has no Internet connection.

The server room can only be accessed by people who are authorised to work with the data or the people that take care of the servers, backups etc. Backups are stored in a safe place such as on an encrypted hard disc, that is in turn stored in a safe place.

The researchers work with the data have all signed the confidentiality agreement, which is the same type that the health personnel working at hospitals have signed.

Possible encryption systems to use are TrueCrypt or Veracrypt[1] both can be executed in Windows, Linux and Mac OS X; however, TrueCrypt is not maintained any more.

9.4 Automatic De-Identification of Patient Records

At Stockholm University for the infrastructure HEALTH BANK—Swedish Health Record Research Bank, the patient records are anonymised in the sense that the tables in the database containing personal names and personal identity numbers

[1] https://veracrypt.codeplex.com. Accessed 2018-01-11.

have been replaced with serial numbers so each individual can be tracked (Dalianis et al. 2015). However this is not really enough for de-identification purposes since plenty of sensitive information resides in the free text in the form of personal names, addresses, telephone numbers etc.

This sensitive information in patient record text is also called Protected Health Information (PHI). In the USA, for example, and many other countries there are requirements that all information in a patient record should be de-identified before the research can be carried out.

The secondary use of these records demands privacy preserving measures. Specifically, it is valuable to know the number, type and nature of fields the sensitive information where present in the electronic patient record.

The American Health Insurance Portability and Accountability Act (HIPAA) (2003), stated which protected health information (PHI) should be removed or obscured from an electronic patient record before the patient record can be used for research. It specifies 18 different PHI classes, such as *personal names, addresses, phone numbers, email addresses, dates, ages over 89, social security numbers*, etc. Note that HIPAA does not require changes to ages under 90 years, institutions or initials.

There have been many attempts to construct de-identification tools, see Uzuner et al. (2007) and Meystre et al. (2010) for nice review articles of different systems. The de-identification systems use both rule-based approaches and machine learning approaches to perform the de-identification, in some cases they use a hybrid approach.

The performance of the systems presented in Meystre et al. (2010) and Uzuner et al. (2007), had F-scores ranging from 0.80 up to, in some cases, 0.97. High recall is preferred over high precision since it is important to identify all sensitive data. Dates and phone numbers obtain the highest scores in de-identification (using rule-based systems or regular expressions), while personal names and in some cases locations obtain lower scores.

For Swedish, Kokkinakis and Thurin (2007) constructed a rule-based system and obtained 96.7% precision, 89.35% recall and obtained an F-score of 0.93. A machine learning-based approach by Dalianis and Velupillai (2010b) utilising Stanford NER CRF and the manually annotated Stockholm EPR PHI Corpus as training and evaluation data yielded an F-score of 0.80. Henriksson et al. (2017b) improved the results on the same data. The authors used extracted features jointly with the CRF to build a predictive model applied on a larger clinical corpus. IOB-encoding of class labels was used, indicates whether a token is inside (I), outside (O) or at the beginning (B), a given named entity in the text. For the feature optimisation L1 and L2 regularisation were used. The best results obtained were 92.65% for precision, 81.29% for recall and an F-score of 0.87.

In production systems both an automatic approach for de-identification and a manual inspection is carried out before the corpus is released for research.

In a recent study by Meystre et al. (2017) the authors have made an extensive review of the status of clinical data reuse and secondary use.

9.4.1 Density of PHI in Electronic Patient Record Text

Regarding the density of PHI in the free text of patient records we can observe the studies such as Douglass et al. (2004). They used MIMIC II, which is a well-known database of patient records and found 1776 instances of PHI in 339,150 tokens giving 0.5% sensitive information in the clinical text.

Dorr et al. (2006) found 1074 instances of PHI in 70,552 tokens, giving 2.9% sensitive information including 1% personal names. The also looked at the different professions and their contribution to the density of PHI, see Table 9.1. One interesting observation is that one human annotator averaged 13,100 tokens and 326 PHI elements per hour.

One well cited work is by Neamatullah et al. (2008) using part of the MIMIC II database. The clinical text consists of 2434 nursing notes containing 334,000 words and 1779 instances of PHI, giving 0.5% PHI. Their manual annotation rate was 18,000 words and 90 PHI terms per hour. The source code and data is available for use.

In Uzuner et al. (2008) is described 889 de-identified discharge summaries in the so-called challenge corpus containing in total 472,315 tokens and 28,188 PHI or 6% of the total data.

The studies mentioned were all for English clinical text, for other languages such as Swedish, Danish and French we have the following studies:

For Swedish clinical text Kokkinakis and Thurin (2007) extracted 14,000 tokens from 200 hospital discharge letters containing 1450 instances of PHI, or 10% of the total amount of text. Velupillai et al. (2009) annotated 174,000 tokens in a Swedish clinical text and found one third was personal names. In total 4423 instances of PHI were found equating 2.5% PHI of the total amount of tokens.

This corpus is also called the Stockholm EPR PHI Corpus and contains 100 patient records from five different clinical units: *neurology, orthopaedia, infection, dental surgery* and *nutrition* (Velupillai et al. 2009), see Table 9.2 for the distribution of PHI entities.

A large amount of the information in an electronic patient record system is unstructured in form of free text. The Stockholm EPR PHI corpus contained

Table 9.1 Authorship of PHI distributed over professions, part of Table 3 in Dorr et al. (2006) for some reason the results add up to over 100%. The authors do not report if these results are normalised according to text size or not

Profession	Percentage PHI
Physician or extender	67.6
Nurse	20.6
Pharmacist	8.0
Social worker	3.4
Other	3.8
Sum	**103.4**

Table 9.2 Types and numbers of annotated tokens in the Stockholm EPR PHI Corpus

Entity	Number of PHI-instances
First name	923
Last name	929
Age	56
Health care unit	1021
Location	148
Full date	500
Date part	710
Phone number	136
Sum	**4423**

380,000 tokens, of these 174,000 tokens were free text giving 46% unstructured information and 54% structured information. The structured information did not include X-rays, images etc. The term, token and word are here used interchangeable. Tokens may also include interpunctuations (Velupillai et al. 2009). The amount of text in the patient records varies depending on the domain studied, for example, psychiatric patient records tend to contain much more text than emergency or general practitioner's records.

For Danish clinical text a study by Pantazos et al. (2016)[2] involved the annotation of 369 full patient records which contained 73,150 words and 1320 instances of PHI, in total 1.8% PHI.

For French clinical text one study by Grouin and Névéol (2014) was performed, annotating 29,437 tokens containing 3964 PHI or 13.4% PHI of which 41% were personal names.

In Hanauer et al. (2013) there is an illustrative heat map visualising and comparing the prevalence of PHI in different document types. In total 116,000 clinical documents written in American English were studied. The study included bootstrapping and pre-annotation to make annotation faster. The highest amount of PHI are in *discharge summaries, outpatient consult, admission history and physical* and *social work notes* overall; dates, clinician and patient personal names were found to have the highest density. In one subset with 20,500 tokens, 752 PHI instances were annotated (in 1 h) giving 3.7% PHI.

Carrell et al. (2013) studied oncology reports found 343 PHI in 22,525 words giving 1.5% PHI.

In another study described in Henriksson et al. (2017b) Swedish patient records were studied, and the highest density of PHI was found in discharge notes written by physicians, and specifically in oncology. The type of PHI that was most prevalent were dates, and first and last names (surnames) of the patient. On average 1.57% PHI was found in the corpus, see Fig. 9.1. In Henriksson et al. (2017a) the trained model were used on other sub corpora, but the performance dropped, probably due

[2]This book is written in memory of Kostas Pantazos who passed away at a young age in October 2015.

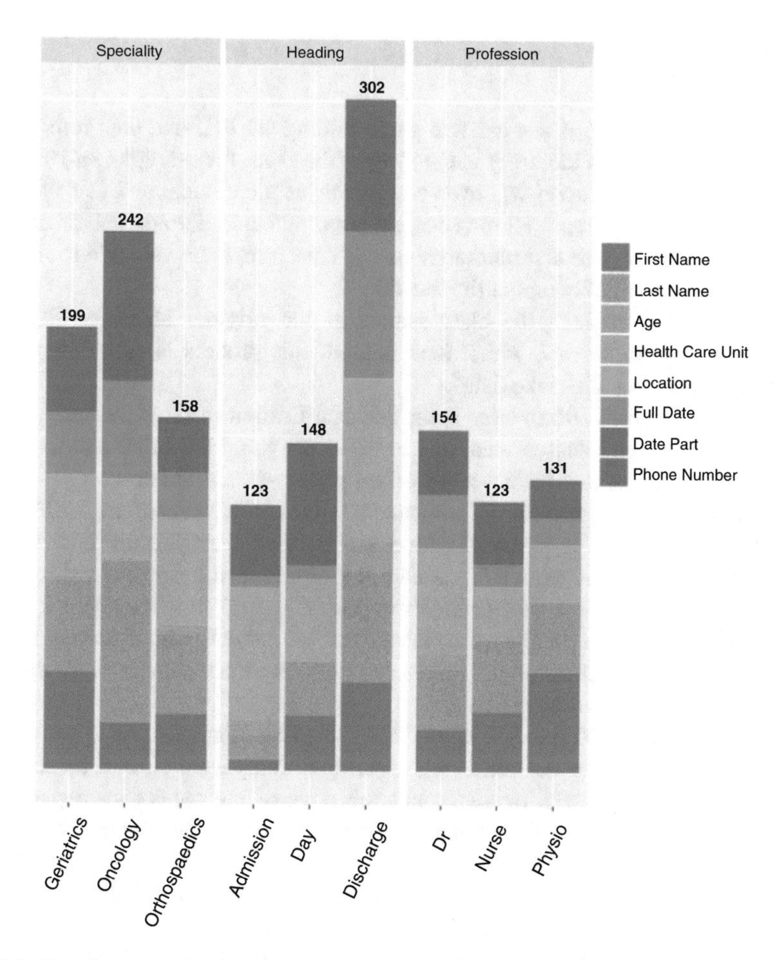

Fig. 9.1 Prevalance and distribution of PHI in various types of clinical notes in HEALTH BANK. Taken from Figure 1 in Henriksson et al. (2017b) (© 2017 The authors—reprinted with permission from the authors and AMIA. Published in Henriksson et al. 2017b)

to the differences in text style. Domain adaption techniques are therefore necessary when training a de-identification system in one domain and processing clinical text from another domain.

The Stockholm EPR PHI Corpus was used for training and the newly annotated *Stockholm EPR PHI Domains Corpus* was used for evaluation. The Stockholm EPR PHI Domains Corpus encompasses the clinical domains *geriatrics, oncology* and *orthopaedics* (including surgery) and contains 1579 annotated instances of PHI: in total there are 63,417 tokens in the corpora. Regarding the Stockholm EPR PHI corpus see Table 9.2.

9.4.2 Pseudonymisation of Electronic Patient Records

The de-identification process has two parts: finding the PHI and then removing or replacing them with an identifier in the form of the class, for example, *patient name, telephone number* or *location*; however, this makes the clinical text less natural to read. Another issue is that PHI may contain important epidemiological information, such as locations where disorders may occur; therefore, is be valuable to maintain some general information about the location.

It is better to replace the class names or the original identified PHI with *surrogates* or *pseudonyms*, which look natural, this process is called *resynthesis* or "re-identification with fake data".

The first attempts to do so were in the de-identification work by Sweeney (1996), where two modules were created, one to de-identify and the other one to replace PHI with surrogates, or what Sweeney called *pseudo-values* in her work.

Each detection algorithm is associated with a replacement algorithm. The strategy is that a date is replaced with a similar date nearby, a personal name is replaced by a fictitious name. These names are produced by orthographical rules creating fictitious names that sounds reasonable but do not belong to a known person. A unique name is always replaced with the same fictitious unique name, a so-called consistent replacement. Sweeney (1996) does not mention how she deals with locations, phone numbers etc.

Douglass et al. (2004) describe how after identification PHI was replaced with surrogates according to the following algorithm: dates were shifted by the same random number of weeks or years, but the days of the weeks were preserved; personal names were replaced with names from the publicly available list of names from the Boston area in the US by randomly substituting first and last names. Locations were replaced by randomly selected small towns; hospitals and hospitals wards were given fictitious names. Moreover, Douglass et al. (2004) explain the process and show the interface of manually validating and correcting the results of the automatic identification and replacement of PHI with surrogates, with the aim of making the corpus available to other researchers.

For Swedish there is a pseudonymisation study by Alfalahi et al. (2012), where personal names are replaced with other personal names in a consistent way, female first names are replaced with common female first names and corresponding is carried out for male first names. Misspelled first names or gender neutral first names are replaced with other gender neutral names, such as *Kim, Pat, Robin* or *Andrea*. Addresses and phone numbers are also replaced, dates are shifted and ages changed slightly. However, locations and healthcare units are replaced by the default location and healthcare unit *Stockholm* and *Solvillan* respectively.

Another study was carried out on the same Swedish data by Antfolk and Branting (2016), where replacement of locations was the focus. The authors replaced locations, such as *places, cities*, and *countries*, with locations that were situated close by to keep possible epidemiological relations, but as the authors also stated there were problems with misspelled or abbreviated locations. Also when a complete address was tagged with *street, street number* and *city*, they did not change it, since this type of pattern was not in the scope of the study. Prepositions before countries could be a problem in some cases. In Swedish the preposition *i* (English: in) and *på* (English: on) could make the replacement of a country name peculiar in some cases. You live on islands, *på Island* (on Iceland) but you live in countries *i Norge* (in Norway).

In a similar study by Björkegren (2011) location was also automatically replaced by surrogates according to the classes: *countries, cities, streets* and *companies/organisations*, since there is only one annotated class called *location* in the de-identified data, each sub class had to be identified using name lists. An evaluation was carried out where three respondents had to decide which of 17 patient records were pseudonymised or an original record. Half of the records were identified as pseudonymised. This concludes the pseudonymisation program was not good enough and the data was still too complicated for natural pseudonymisation. Natural pseudonymisation needs to have consistent geographical information, such as for example that a street is situated in the correct part of the city. This concludes also that more research work has to be carried out, encompassing better annotation work.

In another approach for pseudonymisation for English by Deleger et al. (2014), the authors used the American English clinical corpus from Physionet, i2b2 and the Cincinnati Children's Hospital Medical Center (CCHMC) corpus for *cross-training*[3] and evaluation of their de-identification algorithm. Part of the research work consisted of creating a replacement algorithm for the identified PHI. Dates were replaced with dates in the same format. Telephone area codes were replaced with other existing area codes. The rest of the phone number was replaced with the same number of random numbers. E-mail addresses were replaced with a random set of characters corresponding to the original number of letters. No replaced PHI had any resemblance with any other PHI occurring in the whole dataset. Personal names were replaced with real names originating from the US Census Bureau, with a frequency above 144 (or 0.002% of the data). Gender of the first name was of course considered. Locations such as streets and places were replaced with new random locations from the corpus, and street numbers were replaced with a random number of same length. No combination of street and number reoccurred as in the original corpus.

In a study by Carrell et al. (2013) the authors describe how to hide non-identified PHI, so-called *residual identifiers*, with the method *Hiding In Plain Sight (HIPS)*, which actually involves to removal of annotation on all de-identified PHI, after replacing them with surrogates. This method hides from plain sight the PHI that could not be de-identified, or residual identifiers. Since neither the de-identification system or the human annotators identify the PHI, the secondary users of the de-identified text believe that identified PHI already has replaced by the pseudonymisation system.

---

[3]Training on one corpus and evaluating on the other corpus.

State of the art de-identification systems reach recall rates of 95–97%, by using the technique described in Carrell et al. (2013) 90% of the residual identifiers can be effectively concealed the HIPS without improving the de-identification system. The main point is that the risk can be calculated on re-identifying residual identifiers depending on what class of PHI they belong to. For example, ages, dates and organisation names are more difficult to re-identify than personal names.

Meystre (2015) has written a nice overview of the whole process of de-identification and resynthesis.

9.4.3 Re-Identification and Privacy

There is no 100% guarantee that individuals in a de-identified and resynthesised patient record cannot be identified. However, some experiments have been carried out to test this. Meystre et al. (2014) did an experiment that after de-identification and resynthesis (replacing the PHI with realistic surrogates) of 86 discharge summaries let the treating physician try to identify their patient. The physician had written the discharge summary between 1 and 3 months before the study. Of the five physicians in the study none could identify their patient.

Sweeney (2002) writes about something that is today called *privacy preserving data linkage*, whereby adding more and more data sources to a de-identified database may cause re-identification of individuals. An example of this presented in the study was the governor of the state of Massachusetts, who like many other US state employees had filed his medical record for health insurance. The data was considered to be anonymous and was given out for research, but using another database with voter registration for Cambridge, Massachusetts, the governor could be identified using ZIP code, birth date and gender in both databases.

Sweeney (2002) presents her algorithm called *k-anonymity*. In short, it can calculate the risk of data can being de-identified by counting the number of attributes in a database to conclude if it is safe to link the data or not to the database. As she writes in the article: *A release provides k-anonymity protection if the information for each person contained in the release cannot be distinguished from at least k−1 individuals whose information also appears in the release.*

Gkoulalas-Divanis et al. (2014) compare 45 different algorithms for calculating privacy preserving linkage. The 45 algorithms are divided into two privacy models. One model is used for demographics and the other model is used for diagnosis codes. Furthermore, Gkoulalas-Divanis et al. (2014) discuss two models for data access. One is the protected data repository model where researchers can interact with the aggregated data with some restrictions. The other model is data publishing where the user has complete access to the data.

El Emam et al. (2015) there is a nice description of the three sensitivity levels of data: non-public, quasi public, public data, and the risk for identification; however, they do not mention clinical text explicitly.

Andersen et al. (2014) have a description on how to use distributed sources of patient records for statistical analysis and still preserve privacy using a large set of possible secure multi-party computation algorithms and computing graphs.

Black Box Approach

One approach was considered in the master's thesis of Almgren and Pavlov (2016), also published in Almgren et al. (2016). We can call it the *black box approach*, since the electronic patient records were not directly accessed by the authors. Almgren and Pavlov had knowledge of the format of the sensitive manually annotated data in the electronic patient records to be evaluated, in this case clinical entities in Swedish (disorder & finding, pharmaceutical drug and body structure).

The authors trained two models, word-vectors and a recurrent neural network model, on out of domain (non-clinical) training data using Swedish scientific medical text (Läkartidningen). The program code and the trained models were sent to an authorised person with access to the sensitive data in the black box. The person executed the program code and delivered the numerical results in the form of precision, recall and F-score to the authors, hence the researchers could use the clinical data without ethical permission.

Another interesting approach similar to the black box approach is to remove the free text of the patient records and only keep the features of the tokens, for example, the length of a token, whether the token contains numerical characters, or upper or lowercase characters, POS tags, features of the tokens preceding and following the token to be analysed, and if the token is PHI and what type of PHI. Using this information as features in the Random Forest algorithm gave almost as good results in identifying PHI as using CRF with the same features and the real text (Dalianis and Boström 2012). Hence, the approach by Dalianis and Boström (2012), can be used to release a large amount of sensitive data without a risk of revealing the identity of any patient. Such data can be used to train and evaluate the machine learning system as well as to construct commercial systems.

9.5 Summary of Ethics and Privacy of Patient Records for Clinical Text Mining Research

This chapter has described the process of getting access to electronic patient records for clinical text mining, which includes writing an ethical permission application, removing sensitive information (PHI) such as personal names, phone numbers, addresses etc. in the patient records, getting access to the data and keeping it in a safe storage.

The best automatic de-identification systems obtain an F-scores up to 0.97, but also require manual review before the data can be released for research. Generally, the highest density of sensitive PHI is in the assessment and social fields, and in the discharge summaries of the patient records. On average 2% of the information found in clinical text is sensitive.

Various methods and results for pseudonymisation, meaning the replacement of real PHI with surrogates in electronic records were described.

Another approach, the black box approach, was described where the sensitive text is stored in a protected black box that can be used by external users without direct access to the data.

Finally, was privacy preserving data linkage explained. There is a risk when connecting de-identified data with external databases since it may reveal sensitive hidden information, to avoid this risk privacy preserving data linkage can be used.

Chapter 10
Applications of Clinical Text Mining

This chapter will present the state of the art for a number of applications of clinical text mining such as detection and prediction of healthcare associated infections (HAI), detection of adverse drug events (ADE), followed by resources for adverse drug event detection and continuing with an application of automatic assignment and validation of ICD-10 diagnosis codes. An application of automatic mapping of ICD-10 diagnosis codes to SNOMED CT will also be presented. This chapter then continues with automatic summarisation of patient record, simplification of patient records text and natural language generation of patient record text. Techniques for searching and retrieving patients from patient records for cohort studies are described, and finally some classic systems in medical decision support such as MYCIN are reviewed. Finally an overview of IBM Watson Health is provided.

10.1 Detection and Prediction of Healthcare Associated Infections (HAIs)

This section explains what a healthcare associated infection (HAI) is, why it is important to monitor and predict them and how to do it automatically using the information from the electronic patient records. The performance of systems for detecting HAIs will be compared. This section will also describe in what extent and where such surveillance systems for detecting HAIs are used in practice and commercially.

10.1.1 Healthcare Associated Infections (HAIs)

Healthcare associated infections (HAIs) are plaguing healthcare with suffering patients and heavy costs for society. Healthcare associated infections are also called *hospital associated infections* or *nosocomial infections*.

H. Dalianis, *Clinical Text Mining*, https://doi.org/10.1007/978-3-319-78503-5_10

HAI is defined in Ducel et al. (2002) as:

> An infection acquired in hospital by a patient who was admitted for a reason other than that infection (1). An infection occurring in a patient in a hospital or other health care facility in whom the infection was not present or incubating at the time of admission. This includes infections acquired in the hospital but appearing after discharge, and also occupational infections among staff of the facility (2).

It is estimated that 10% of all in-patients will obtain a healthcare associated infection while treated for another disorder (Humphreys and Smyth 2006). It is estimated that in Europe there are three million affected patients per year, of which about 50,000 die. The lethal outcome seems dramatic, but many of these patients had severe disorders, or multiple disorders, were old and had been treated at the hospital for a longer period of time and would have died of the disease, but the HAI hastened their death.

In Sweden with a population of 10 million the expected yearly cost for HAIs is estimated as 6.5 billion SEK or approximately 800 million USD. This cost corresponds to 750,000 extra days in hospital (SALAR 2014).

An important goal in defeating HAIs is to collect statistics by detecting and measure the prevalence of HAIs, but also to predict and warn if a particular patient has a high risk of obtaining HAI. HAIs can encompass, for example, pneumonia, urinary tract infection, sepsis or various wound infections but also norovirus (winter vomiting disease).

Part of the definition of HAI is that the patient must have been admitted to the hospital for more than 48 h before an infection can be defined as a HAI. The patient can also have been admitted and discharged then re-admitted to the same hospital (or to another hospital) within 24 h, as long as the patient entire healthcare period episode lasted more than 48 h the definition of HAI remains valid, see Fig. 10.1.

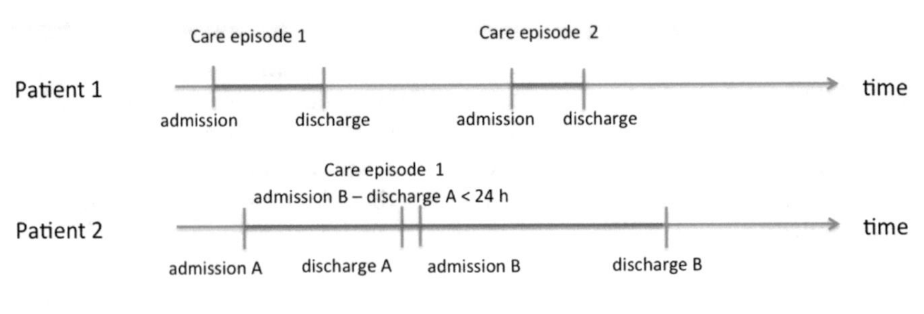

Fig. 10.1 If a patient (Patient 2) is discharged from one clinical unit and admitted to another within 24 h and the whole period is more than 48 h then that patient is considered to be admitted for the whole care episode and can therefore be analysed for HAIs. This figure is courtesy of Hideyuki Tanushi (© 2014 Springer International Publishing Switzerland—reprinted with permission. Published in Dalianis (2014))

To detect and predict HAI, the *healthcare episodes* of the patient record are used. Healthcare (or care) episodes are the daily notes and data that are entered into the patient record regarding the treatment and status of the patient. By observing the information in the care episodes a picture can be obtained whether the patient has a high risk of obtaining a HAI or not, or if the patient has obtained a HAI.

In Sweden a HAI must be reported by law, unfortunately, that is not always the case. Sometimes the reporting is not carried out because of ignorance and sometimes because physicians treating a patient for lethal diseases such as cancer or rheumatism are focusing on curing the patient and not on reporting the HAI. The physician believes that the HAI is just a small side effect or obstacle on the path to cure the patient of a much more serious disease.

One issue is how underreported are HAIs? To solve this problem, the National Board of Health and Welfare in Sweden (Socialstyrelsen) requires that all hospitals in Sweden report how many in-patients in each clinical unit have HAIs on one specific day. This measurement is carried out twice a year, once in the fall and once in the spring. This measurement is called the Point Prevalence Measurement (PPM). By performing the PPM the authorities can obtain an indication of how many patients have a HAI at each clinical unit, on each hospital, 24 h a day throughout Sweden; however, since the PPM is only carried out twice a year and does not give all the information needed, the hospital management would like to have continuous measurement with more measurement points every day and year round.

If specific measure are taken to avoid HAIs, for example, the use of new antibacterial catheters, special equipment in the ward, new cleaning routines for the ward, or single rooms for the patients, then it would be valuable to automatically measure the effect by using the daily nursing notes and doctor notes as input to a HAI monitoring system.

10.1.2 Detecting and Predicting HAI

An automatic HAI detection system analyses the text and the structured information in the patient record for specific terms that may point to a HAI. Such terms may be specific antibiotics for treating HAIs, particular microbiological tests for typical HAI bacteria as well as high body temperatures indicating infection. Risk prone patients are patients with catheters that are present in the body for a long time, patients that have been operated on and patients with open wounds along with generally older patients who stay on a ward for a long time.

There have been many approaches for detecting HAIs using only the structured information in the patient records, or the clinical free text, or both the structured information and the clinical text. Both rule-based methods and machine learning-based methods have been used. The best system obtained up to 97% precision and recall. Usually high recall is more important than high precision in detecting HAI. For a nice review of different HAI detecting systems or HAI surveillance systems see Freeman et al. (2013).

Table 10.1 Statistics for the Stockholm EPR Detect-HAI Corpus

	HAI	non-HAI
Number of records	128	85
Patient ages [years]	2–93	2–92
Total number of tokens	1,034,760	230,226
Time in hospital [days]	2–144	3–93
Total time in hospital [days]	3975	941

Tokens refer to space separated sequences of characters

Proux et al. (2011) describe a rule-based system for detection of HAIs in French patient records called *Assitant de Lutte Automatise et de Detection des Infections Nosocomiales a partir de Documents Textuels Hospitaliers (ALADIN-DTH)*, or simply ALADIN.

Ehrentraut et al. (2014) present a machine learning-based system called Detect-HAI for Swedish patient records using the *Stockholm EPR Detect-HAI Corpus*, see Table 10.1.

Two machine learning algorithms Support Vector Machine (SVM) and Random Forest (RF) in the Weka toolkit were applied on the annotated Stockholm EPR Detect-HAI Corpus. The corpus were preprocessed using nine different preprocessing steps were carried out including NegEx to detect negated expressions in the clinical text, however the preprocessing step that gave the best result was lemmatisation jointly with the Random Forest algorithm that gave 87% recall and 83% precision and an F-score of 0.85 (Ehrentraut et al. 2014).

The results using the same corpus were improved by utilising the Gradient Tree Boosting (GTB) algorithm in the Scikit-learn toolkit, obtaining 93.7% recall and 79.7% precision and F-score of 85.7 (Ehrentraut et al. 2016).

An approach using deep learning to detect HAI also studied the same data, the Stockholm EPR Detect-HAI Corpus, was carried out in (Jacobson and Dalianis 2016). The best results were obtained using the stacked restricted Boltzmann machines with a recall of 88% and with a precision of 79%. The results were comparable to those obtained in Ehrentraut et al. (2014); however, they were slightly lower than the results presented in Ehrentraut et al. (2016). Probably the annotated used data in the study was too sparse to make full use of the power of deep learning algorithms that require a large amount of annotated data.

Another general problem with the Stockholm EPR Detect-HAI Corpus presented in Table 10.1 is that the normal distribution of HAI and non-HAI data is 10 to 90 (around 10% of all patients have a HAI) while the distribution in the Stockholm EPR Detect-HAI Corpus is 60 to 40; hence, it does not reflect the real situation.

A rule-based approach using Swedish clinical text to detect urinary tract infections was investigated by Tanushi et al. (2014), both the data and text of the patient record were used. The data was divided in care episodes according to Fig. 10.2. (The same input data was used for the machine learning approaches of Ehrentraut et al. (2016) and Jacobson and Dalianis (2016)).

For the development of these systems, two development sets were used; one that had been used for the PPM containing 100 patient records and their corresponding

```
123 H - IVA 322916614D 2007-08-21 9:12 1944 Woman
Anamnesis
Got a urine catheter two days ago. Done a lab test
on the urine and gave antibiotics.
<ICD-10 code>
I110 Pneumonia.
I509 Heart failure, unspecified.

<Current medication>
Penomax

<Body temperature>
38
38
38.5

123 H - IVA 322916614D 2007-08-22 16:12 1944 Woman
<Body temperature>
37
36.8
36.9

<Blood culture>
pseudomonas
```

Fig. 10.2 An example of an electronic patient record text translated to English. The text is in a format prepared for processing by a computer program for detecting HAIs. The important features are extracted from the patient record and the program can check the status of a patient day by day. This particular patient got HAI (© 2014 Springer International Publishing Switzerland—reprinted with permission. Published in Dalianis (2014))

215 care episodes from different clinical units, and the other one containing 66 patient records from a rheumatology unit and their corresponding 134 care episodes. Both development sets were assessed for HAI and non-HAI by two physicians, one of them a specialist in infectious diseases.

For the evaluation 1195 patient records from oncological and surgical clinical units corresponding to 1867 care episodes with a duration ranging from 2 to 14 days were used. The resulting rule-based system obtained 98% precision and 60% recall. Observe that the evaluated results are from a different domain than the development of the system.

10.1.3 Commercial HAI Surveillance Systems and Systems in Practical Use

There are many different HAI surveillance systems in use worldwide, most of them use the structured information in the patient record, however, some of them use the clinical free text in addition to the structured data. Most systems are in-house developed systems and not commercial systems (Freeman et al. 2013).

In Sweden, the Anti-Infection tool, (Infektionsverktyget)[1] is used at all hospitals, it is integrated with each electronic patient record system. The Anti-Infection tool forces the prescribing physician at the hospital to state whether antibiotics are prescribed to a patient for prophylactic reasons, for an infection acquired outside the healthcare facility or for a healthcare associated infection. This information is collected nationwide and statistics are produced; however, it only tracks healthcare associated infections that are known and infections that can be treated by antibiotics.

One third of the hospitals in California, USA, use automated surveillance technology (AST) to monitor HAI. Some of the systems use information from the text in the patient record as well. The AST systems are a mix of in-house produced parts and commercially delivered parts (Halpin et al. 2011). Halpin et al. (2011) conclude that there is a strong and statistically significant association of the use of AST and evidence-based practice[2] for the prevention of HAI.

Monitoring of Nosocomial Infections in Intensive Care Units (MONI-ICU) is a surveillance system for electronic patient records written in German, using both text and data. MONI-ICU is used at the Vienna General Hospital in Austria as well as several other hospitals in Germany (Blacky et al. 2011). MONI-ICU has obtained a sensitivity (recall) of 90% and a specificity of 100% for intensive care unit patient records.

Testing of the French ALADIN system has been carried out in four French University hospitals (Lille, Lyon, Nice and Rouen), but has not yet implemented in practice (Proux et al. 2011; Metzger et al. 2012).

10.2 Detection of Adverse Drug Events (ADEs)

Adverse drug events (ADEs) are a major public health problem, around 5% of all hospital admissions in the world are due to ADEs (Beijer and de Blaey 2002). In Sweden, the seventh most common cause of death is an ADE (Wester et al. 2008). The domain of detection of adverse drug events (ADEs), is a complicated area. The relation between the properties of the body of a particular person, the disorder the person has and the pharmacological properties of the drug need to be understood. All drugs are poisonous in some sense but given in the correct amount they may cure a disease.

[1]The Anti-Infection Tool, http://www.inera.se/Documents/TJANSTER_PROJEKT/Infektionsverktyget/The_AntiInfection_tool.pdf. Accessed 2018-01-11.

[2]Evidence-based medicine is a concept within medicine meaning that the treatment of the patient should follow scientific results from well-designed research.

10.2.1 Adverse Drug Events (ADEs)

The science concerning drug safety is called pharmacovigilance or sometimes drug safety surveillance, and is related to the collection, detection, assessment, monitoring and prevention of adverse effects.

According to the World Health Organisation (WHO) the definition of an adverse drug reaction (ADR) is *a response to a drug that is noxious and unintended and occurs at doses normally used in man for the prophylaxis, diagnosis or therapy of disease, or for modification of physiological function* (Edwards and Aronson 2000).

An adverse effect can be in a range of severity from very mild to very strong, even lethal, and of various types. Usually an *adverse drug effect* is seen from the view of the drug while an *adverse reaction* is seen from the view of the patient.

There are six types of adverse effects (Edwards and Aronson 2000):

(a) *Dose-related*, for example giving toxic effect.
(b) *Non-dose related*, for example penicillin hypersensitivity.
(c) *Dose-related and time-related*, related to the cumulative dose.
(d) *Time-related*, becomes apparent some time after the use of the drug.
(e) *Withdrawal*, occurs after the withdrawal of the drug.
(f) *Unexpected*, often caused by drug interactions.

When the pharmaceutical industry is developing new drugs, at an early stage in the development the drug is tested on humans, usually on healthy young men to study how the human body is affected by the drug and also to detect possible adverse drug effects, while most patients taking a drug are older and suffering from some disorder and, of course, half of them are women. Drugs are usually not tested on women at this stage since women may become pregnant during the tests and the fetus may be affected by the drug.

In other words the sample size for the test is small, the duration of the test is short.

At a second stage the drug is tested on a small group of patients in a so-called *clinical trial* to test the effect of the drug before the drug is approved for the market.

During the clinical trial two test groups of patients are usually created, one is given the drug and the other group, the control group, is given a substitute which does not contain any active ingredients, a *placebo*.

Postmarketing surveillance (PMS) or post market surveillance is carried out to monitor the effect of drugs after they have been released to the market. PMS covers a larger sample over a longer period than a clinical trial.

An adverse drug effect or adverse effect is a general term for all types of unwanted effects of drugs. An adverse drug effect is hopefully mild and probably known by the physician, it is also related to the pharmacological properties of the drug. An adverse drug reaction may also be fatal and probably not known by the physician (Edwards and Aronson 2000; Läkemedelsverket 2012).

In the text mining terminology of adverse drug events the following concepts are used: an *adverse drug event (ADE)* may occur when a drug is taken to treat a disease. The disease may be indicated by a number of symptoms or findings. This is an *indication* for prescribing a drug. A *contraindication* is a factor or reason to cease or withhold the treatment of the patient with the drug, since the it may harm the patient.

The drug treats the disease but the drug may also give the patient an undesired side effect or adverse drug event, a so-called *ADE cause*, in terms of a new finding or a new disorder, this drug reaction is called an *ADE Cue* in our clinical text mining processing vocabulary (Henriksson et al. 2015). Another article describing the terminology in a nice way is written by Nebeker et al. (2004).

Some of ADEs are known, others are not known and hence are called unknown drug events or unknown side effects. Some drugs also interact with other drugs and give undesired effects, so-called *drug-drug interactions* or just *drug interaction*, (some drug-drug interactions can also give a positive effect).

Sometimes a drug is prescribed to remove the adverse drug effect or symptoms of a drug. For example, when a drug is given as chemotherapy to a patient to treat cancer tumors and the patient feels nausea as an adverse drug effect, then another drug may be given to the patient to mitigate the nausea.

The state of the art in drug development is personalised medicine, meaning that each patient should, for example, obtain a customised drug adapted specifically for that individual's genetic properties and corresponding disorder.

10.2.2 Resources for Adverse Drug Event Detection

To detect adverse drug events expressed in textual form and in structured data in the patient record a number of resources are needed.

First of all, ICD-10 diagnosis codes related to adverse drug events that are assigned to the patient records need to be studied, see Table 10.2, for examples. These ICD-10 diagnosis codes are assigned to the discharge summary by the physician if a patient has experienced an ADE, but in many cases in no code assigned even if an ADE has occurred.

Secondly, natural language expressions, indicating ADEs in the clinical text can be studied. In a clinical text when a patient is suffering some form of adverse drug reaction it is expressed by a phrase such as: *drug-induced reaction in form of drug X*, or just *reaction, hypersensitivity* or *adverse reaction*, it can also be vague or uncertain expressions such as *suspected hypersensitivity*, or *possible reaction on drug*. Expressions similar to these have been extracted from Swedish clinical text by human annotators (Friedrich and Dalianis 2015; Henriksson et al. 2015). The adverse event cues in Swedish used in Friedrich and Dalianis (2015) can be found on the DSV website.[3]

[3] Adverse event cues in Swedish from Friedrich and Dalianis (2015), see under *Swedish ADE word lists* in http://dsv.su.se/health/tools. Accessed 2018-01-11.

Table 10.2 ICD-10 diagnosis codes for adverse drug events

ICD-10 code	Description
E27.3	Drug-induced adrenocortical insufficiency
G24.0	Drug induced dystonia
G25.1	Drug-induced tremor
G44.4	Drug-induced headache, not elsewhere classified
G62.0	Drug-induced polyneuropathy
I42.7	Cardiomyopathy due to drug and external agent
I95.2	Hypotension due to drugs
L27.0	Generalized skin eruption due to drugs and medicaments taken internally
L27.1	Localized skin eruption due to drugs and medicaments taken internally
N14.1	Nephropathy induced by other drugs, medicaments and biological substances
T78.2	Anaphylactic shock, unspecified
T78.3	Angioneurotic edema
T80.8	Other complications following infusion, transfusion and therapeutic injection
T88.7	Unspecified adverse effect of drug or medicament
T88.6	Anaphylactic reaction due to adverse effect of correct drug or medicament properly administered

The table is taken from Table 1 in Henriksson et al. (2015). Licensed under Creative Commons

Another way to find typical expressions is to use *Farmaceutiska Specialiteter i Sverige (FASS)*, the Swedish corresponding list of the American *PDR, Physician's Desk Reference*. FASS contains all drugs on the market in Sweden and is written for physicians, nurses, dentists and all clinicians allowed to prescribe drugs in Sweden. FASS listed each drug name, pharmacological property, ATC-code and which type of adverse reaction a drug may give, along with the probability of this. To use these terms, it is necessary to download them.

The same information can be extracted from the search tool at *Läkemedelsverket*[4] and, the API[5] and the open data for drugs can be found online.[6] The data in XML format is also available.[7]

The terms used for side effects are often very general and can not really be connected to a particular drug. Resource for performing text mining research for detecting adverse drug events is the *WHO Adverse Reactions Terminology (WHO-ART)*.[8]

[4]Läkemedelsverket, the Swedish Medical Products Agency, drug search tool (in Swedish), https://lakemedelsverket.se/LMF/. Accessed 2018-01-11.

[5]API, http://lakemedelsboken.se/api/. Accessed 2018-01-11.

[6]Open data (in Swedish), https://lakemedelsverket.se/psidata. Accessed 2018-01-11.

[7]XML, https://npl.mpa.se/mpa.npl.services/home2.aspx. Accessed 2018-01-11.

[8]WHO-ART, http://www.umc-products.com/DynPage.aspx?id=73589&mn1=1107&mn2=1664. Accessed 2018-01-11.

If a more fine grained terminology is needed the *Medical Dictionary for Regulatory Activities (MedDRA)* can be used.[9]

10.2.3 Passive Surveillance of ADEs

Postmarketing adverse drug surveillance is important, but is mainly carried out spontaneously by sending a report to the *Uppsala Monitoring Centre (UMC)*[10] when an adverse event has occurred. (UMC is a WHO collaborating centre for international drug monitoring).

Postmarketing adverse drug surveillance is also called *passive surveillance*. However, many physicians consider some ADEs as well known and unavoidable while treating the patient for a more serious, may be lethal disease. Therefore, new methods are needed to perform postmarketing adverse drug surveillance, one method is, for example, to use the large repositories of electronic patient records, both the structured and the unstructured part. The patient records may contain typical patterns of ADEs and undertaking a statistical and register-based data analysis may reveal new or unknown events (Jensen et al. 2012; Harpaz et al. 2012).

10.2.4 Active Surveillance of ADEs

The concept of *adverse event alerting systems*, is using patient data and to analyse adverse event has occurred, this method is also called *Active surveillance*. In a nice review article by Forster et al. (2012), over 48 systems were compared, the earliest from 1988 and the latest from 2008; however, it is not clear exactly how the alerting systems work. The review article mentions rules and a gold standard but it is not clear how the input data is formatted, whether the input data is structured or unstructured. The authors express a wish, in the article, that the systems could also use free-text for the analysis of adverse drug effects. Generally, the different systems presented in the review article, gave rather poor results. The average sensitivity (recall) is around 60% and the average specificity is around 60%, the best system had 94% sensitivity and 71% specificity. The systems are also difficult to compare because they use different input data, but this is a common problem in many applications.

In Bailey et al. (2016) 108 adverse event reporting systems were compared and most of the systems used free-text in the analysis. One finding was that half of the systems had qualitative scores between 60% and 80%, meaning no system had top

[9]MedDRA, http://www.meddra.org. Accessed 2018-01-11.

[10]Uppsala Monitoring Centre, http://who-umc.org. Accessed 2018-01-11.

results and it was also difficult to compare the systems since the input data was different for each system.

In the review article by Warrer et al. (2012) the authors have focused an text mining-based adverse drug alerting systems. Over 200 articles, published from 2001 to 2010, but mainly between 2009 and 2010, were investigated. Seven articles were selected, however the articles presented low specificity and positive value, or precision (PPV), values for the different systems. Warrer et al. (2012) conclude that text mining can only be a supplement to manual chart review for screening large amounts data.

Stausberg and Hasford (2011) carried out a registry study in Germany over the years 2003–2007 using 505 specific ICD-10 codes as definitions for ADEs, the codes were in turn categorised into seven groups depending on the certainty. The finding was that 5% of the hospital episodes were either caused or complicated by an ADE, this is based on approximately 48 million hospital episodes equating to approximately 12 million hospital episodes per year. Similar results were found for the Stockholm EPR Corpus for the years 2009–2010, with 6.6% of the patients having an ADE, calculated on 703,173 patient records (Lagos 2016).

In an extensive article of text and data mining techniques by Karimi et al. (2015b), the authors review the area of ADEs, and also various tools for both data and text mining applied on clinical records and social media to detect ADE.

Another interesting review article in the area of text mining ADEs is by Luo et al. (2017).

10.2.5 Approaches for ADE Detection

To find adverse events, the clinical entities have to be detected, such as *symptom, diagnosis, body part* and *drug*, as well as the relations between the entities.

As previously described, the early approaches in detecting ADEs were rule-based approaches, and the earliest systems did not even analyse the free text but only the structured data.

Here follow some approaches using the textual information as input and a rule-based approach to detect the ADEs.

Eriksson et al. (2013) performed a rule- and dictionary-based approach to detect ADEs in 6011 Danish psychiatric patients' hospital records. The system identified 35,477 unique ADEs with a precision of 0.89 and a recall of 0.75.

Wang et al. (2009) developed a rule-based system to detect the relationship between the drug and the ADEs for seven different types of drugs (ibuprofen, morphine, warfarin, bupropion, paroxetine, rosiglitazone and ACE inhibitors). 25,074 discharge summaries in English were used to evaluate the system. The authors obtained a recall and precision of 0.75 and 0.31 respectively for known ADEs.

Hazlehurst et al. (2009) used the Kaiser Permanente Northwest (KPNW) database containing records for more than 450,000 people to detect vaccine

ADEs. Two automatic methods were compared, the MediClass and the code-based detection. MediClass method obtained better results, than code-based method with 0.74 versus 0.31 PPV (positive predictive value, or precision).

Here follows some machine learning-based approaches for detecting adverse drug events.

Gurulingappa et al. (2012) manually annotated an English corpus containing 3000 medical case reports (i.e. published scientific reports for selected patients with regard to drugs and side effects). The annotation concepts used were *drugs, drug dosage, adverse effect* and their relationship. The corpus was annotated jointly by three annotators, two experienced and one novice annotator in text mining related topics. All of the annotators had an M.Sc. degree in biomedicine.

Each annotator annotated 2000 case reports, and 1000 case reports were annotated by all three annotators. Inter-annotator agreement (IAA) for drugs obtained F-scores for partial match ranging from 0.90 down to 0.38. IAA for relations for drugs-adverse effect obtained F-scores ranging from 0.79 down to 0.37. The ADE-corpus is publicly available.[11]

Naïve-Bayes and Maximum Entropy (MaxEnt) classifiers from the MALLET toolkit were used for training, when evaluated they obtained at best 0.75 precision and 0.64 recall for MaxEnt.

Santiso et al. (2014) studied Spanish clinical text and used 6100 concepts and 4700 adverse drug reactions (ADRs) relations for training using the Random Forest algorithm. 2100 concepts and 1600 ADR relations were used for evaluation, and their Random Forest approach obtained 0.93 precision and 0.85 recall.

Aramaki et al. (2010) used 3012 Japanese discharge summaries containing 1045 drugs and 3601 possible adverse drug effects that were manually annotated. The finding was that 7.7% of the discharge summaries contained ADEs, 59% of these could be extracted automatically. Both support vector machine (SVM) and pattern matching (PTN) methods were used. Marginally better results were obtained using PTN. PTN gave a precision of 0.41 and a recall of 0.92, whereas SVM gave a precision of 0.58 and a recall of 0.62.

Roller and Stevenson (2014) used UMLS to identify concepts, such as drugs and contraindications, and relations, such as ADE drug relations, in millions of biomedical scientific articles. A Naïve-Bayes classifier was trained on the data and 25% precision and 100% recall was obtained.

In another type of approach that is not connected to clinical text mining, but to social media analytics Karimi et al. (2015a) used social media textual posts of patient-reported ADEs to find adverse drug events. The annotated corpus is called the CSIRO Adverse Drug Event Corpus (CADEC).

[11] Benchmark corpus to support information extraction for adverse drug effects, https://sites.google.com/site/adecorpus/. Accessed 2018-01-11.

An Approach for Swedish Clinical Text

The *Clinical Entity Finder (CEF)* (Skeppstedt et al. 2014) was used by Henriksson et al. (2015) to speed up annotation by utilising pre-annotation. *Pre-annotation* means a text is annotated by a machine to assist the human annotator. The model for pre-annotation was trained on annotated records from an internal medicine emergency unit obtained from an earlier annotation study. The records were annotated with the entities *finding, disorder, body structure* and *pharmaceutical drug*.

The clinical text to be annotated was extracted based on the ICD-10 codes indicating ADEs, see Table 10.2 for the specific codes.

The annotations were carried out by three annotators, one junior and one senior computer scientist and one physician. The three annotators corrected both the pre-annotated entities and added missing ones. They also added an annotation for the new entity *ADE cue*. They added optional attributes to the clinical entities *finding, disorder, body part, drug* and *ADE*. Attributes such as *negation, speculation, past* and *future*. Then commenced the difficult part of the annotation work, and which was to draw arches to annotate the indications and also the ADEs. The following semantic relations between named entities were annotated: *indication adverse drug event, ADE outcome* and *ADE cause*.

The agreement for the annotators versus the pre-annotations was high, giving a macro-averaged F-score of 0.825, indicating the pre-annotation model generalises well to a different medical domain.

The inter-annotator agreement was fairly high, above an F-score of 0.8. Lower agreement was found for the class ADE cue, may be due to not being defined properly or because it was mixed up with the classes disorder and finding. In total 3789 named entities, 1642 attributes and 2266 relations were annotated. Bag of Words (BOW), Semantic Vectors (SV) and Multiple Semantic Vectors (MSV) were all used for the text mining; however, the relation mining part produce rather low F-score, the best for SV, being below 0.30. This is probably because the relations cross over several sentences and are difficult to detect.

The PhD thesis by Henriksson (2015) contains a nice approach for using unsupervised learning and ensembles of semantic spaces within random indexing, to produce features used in machine learning to detect ADEs in Swedish clinical text.

In Fig. 6.1 we can see part of the annotation work carried out by Henriksson et al. (2015), which is part of Henriksson's PhD thesis (Henriksson 2015).

An Approach for Spanish Clinical Text

Casillas et al. (2016) developed a system to detect adverse drug reactions (ADRs), for Spanish electronic health records. The patient records were obtained from Galdakao-Usansolo Hospital in Usansolo, Bizkaia, Spain. In total they used 194 patient records containing 101,685 words. The documents were annotated by four experts in pharmacovigilance from the same hospital; however, no inter-annotator agreement results were reported. In total 3084 entities were annotated jointly with 4994 events. The events involve drug-disease pairs where the drug caused the disease, i.e. an adverse drug event including the causal relation.

One remark was that the majority of the relations are inter-sentential, stretching over more than 10 sentences from the disease entity to the drug entity, in the positive ADR event cases. Distance between entities in terms of the number of sentences from the disease entity to the drug entity in the case of positive ADR events was one of the features, other features used were the symptoms lexicon, the drugs lexicon, and keywords between the two lexicons.

One other obvious remark was that there was an imbalance between negative and positive ADR events, where only 6% of the drug-disease entity pairs triggered a positive drug reaction.

The annotated corpus was divided into a training set and a test set. Random Forest, (RF) and Support Vector Machine (SVM) algorithms were used for the training.

In parallel, a rule-based system was also developed as well as a hybrid system using a combination of the rule and machine learning-based approaches.

The rule-based system obtained a rather high precision of 0.89 but a low recall of 0.12, and both the machine learning and the hybrid systems produced poor results, with precision and a recall of less than 0.54.

In the article it also states that the "hospital found the system well worth using, not as an automatic ADR event extraction system but as a decision support system" (Casillas et al. 2016).

A Joint Approach for Spanish and Swedish Clinical Text

Pérez et al. (2017) carried out a joint approach for Spanish and Swedish clinical text to extract disease and drug in Spanish and body part disorder and finding in Swedish using the same methods on different corpora. The methods were maximum probability, CRF, perceptron and SVM. CRF gave the best result on the development sets for both languages and the perceptron the best result on the Spanish test set.

10.3 Suicide Prevention by Mining Electronic Patient Records

Adverse event detection in electronic patient records for suicide risk is an important application for clinical text mining. According to Leonard Westgate et al. (2015) suicide was, in 2010, the tenth leading cause of death in the United States and among the top four leading causes of death for Americans between the ages of 10 and 54.

There have been some early applications in the area of clinical text and data mining in the domain, most approaches have been to perform data mining on the structured information in patient records such as ICD-10 or ICD-9 coding for suicide attempts and self harming (Tran et al. 2014; Barak-Corren et al. 2016).

However, Leonard Westgate et al. (2015) used simple linguistic analysis and Gkotsis et al. (2016) developed a negation detection solution using psychiatric electronic health records for detecting suicide risk.

Haerian et al. (2012) used a combination of ICD-9 coding and UMLS Concept Unique Identifiers for text mining of suicidal expressions in the electronic patient records. The best results they obtained were a positive predictive value (PPV) or precision of 97% with a 90% confidence interval of 0.92–0.99.

Metzger et al. (2016) studied electronic patient records in French from an emergency unit to carry out an epidemiological surveillance study of suicide attempts. The authors used 444 patient records with both recorded suicide attempts and suicidal ideations and 292 patient records as control group, they used the Random Forest and Naïve Bayes machine learning methods obtaining F-scores ranging from 70.4% to 95.3%.

Their study shows that the national manual coding made at the Croix-Rousse Hospital (Red Cross Hospital) were massively underestimated, as the number of events, only 15 of total 98 emergency department visits related to suicide attempts in 2012, were recorded in the national manual coding, while their text mining approach gave adequate results with much less work load for the physicians in the emergency department.

In another study by Downs et al. (2017) 230,465 British English anonymised clinical records were used containing 500 patients with autism spectrum disorders (ASD). The aim of the study was to detect suicide risk in ASD adolescents. The authors used a rule-based NLP approach and obtained high system performance with precision, recall and F-scores of over 0.85 for detecting positive and negative suicidality. Each patient record encompasses a large number of notes over time, it is, therefore, difficult for the annotators to classify whether something is suicide-related or not from only the information in one note.

Moreover, suicide-related terms are very rare in the notes. less that 3%. Another difficulty is that the terms might be references to the past, about other family members, relatives or friends. Suicidal expressions can be very vague, e.g. "took an excessive amount of pills", or very abstract, it can also be as part of a behavioural change of the patient without even explicitly mentioning suicide-related information. These are problems a NLP tool has to overcome as well as the human annotator.

There are still relatively few articles in this domain, using free text in the patient records for suicide risk detection, but hopefully research in this area will increase soon.

10.4 Mining Pathology Reports for Diagnostic Tests

There have been attempts to automatise the process of interpreting, the unstructured text of pathology reports and automatically enter it into the database of the cancer registry, mostly using various text mining tools to extract the diagnostic tests from the pathology text. Part of this work has also involved encouraging pathologists to enter structured information into the pathology report hence making it easier for the text mining tools. A description and overview of various tools is available in Scharber (2007).

The text mining tools for pathology reports are mostly rule-based but there are also some machine learning-based tools, for a review article on the topic, see Spasić et al. (2014) and also Weegar and Dalianis (2015).

Currie et al. (2006) describe a rule-based approach to extract concepts from 5826 breast cancer and 2838 prostate cancer pathology reports. Their system extracted 80 fields and obtained 90–95% accuracy. The system was evaluated by domain experts.

Coden et al. (2009) have written an extensive article on how to extract nine different classes from the pathology free text describing colon cancer using both machine learning and rule-based approaches. Hybrid methods were used in the work by Ou and Patrick (2014). The authors studied pathology reports concerning primary cutaneous melanomas (skin cancer) and extracted 28 different concepts.

Martinez and Li (2011) used machine learning to classify pathology reports for colorectal cancer according to the TNM staging scale. The authors used the Weka toolkit and the algorithms Naïve-Bayes and SVM for the best results. In Nguyen et al. (2011) a rule-based method for mining pathology reports for lung cancer is described.

A study with very good results was carried out by Buckley et al. (2012) on 76,000 breast pathology reports, where they obtained results with 99.1% sensitivity (recall) and 96.5% specificity; however, it is not clear what method they used to extract the information apart from the commercial tool developed by *Clearforest, Waltham, MA*, nor is the method for evaluation of their results explained.

Another study using machine learning on surgical pathology reports for cancer also gave good results with a maximum of 99.4% accuracy using the perceptron algorithm with uneven margins (the PAUM-algorithm). The reports were manually annotated pathology reports in British English. The training set and test set contained 635 and 163 reports respectively. The evaluation used was fivefold cross-validation (Napolitano et al. 2016).

Two studies using machine learning, both for breast cancer pathology reports one for English and one for Chinese were reported in Yala et al. (2017) and in Tang et al. (2018) respectively. Both studies obtained promising results.

10.4.1 The Case of the Cancer Registry of Norway

At the Cancer Registry of Norway (Kreftregisteret) in Oslo over 25 full time experts are manually coding 180,000 pathology reports annually from the whole of Norway which has a population of 5.3 million inhabitants. The pathology reports are written in Norwegian. The experts read the free text in the pathology reports and produce structured coding that is stored jointly with the pathology reports in XML-format. The coding is carried out for research and statistical purposes, and stored in a database.

Three studies will be described here that use the same set of pathology reports from the Cancer Registry of Norway as input data. All three studies use rule-based approaches. One of the studies used a larger data set than the other two.

The first study is by Singh et al. (2015) using 25 pathology reports for prostate cancer written in free text in Norwegian. The authors used the SAS Institute software to extract fields. Their system obtained 76% correctly extracted fields for number of biopsies and 24% for number of biopsies containing tumor tissue, and 100% for Gleason score; however, the study focuses on system development and the evaluation of the system is not described.

The second study is by Dahl et al. (2016) using the same 25 pathology reports for prostate cancer in free text used by Singh et al. (2015). Half of the reports were used as a development set and the other half as a test set. The developed system obtained an F-score of 0.94 on four data points *total malign, primary gleason, secondary gleason* and *total gleason*.

The third study is by Weegar et al. (2017) that used a much larger subset of pathology reports for prostate cancer than used by both Singh et al. (2015) and Dahl et al. (2016). Weegar et al. (2017) built a rule-based system which extracted structured information from over 554 pathology reports for prostate cancer written in Norwegian. The authors divided the 554 pathology reports in 388 documents for the development set and 176 documents for the test set. The system extracts structured information from the free text describing biopsies and Gleason grades. The system obtained an F-score of 0.91. The most interesting part of the system is a flagging mechanism that identifies reports that contain ambiguities or other problems, and therefore need manual review. The system shows the possibility to automatise encoding and make it faster but still with high quality. See Fig. 10.3 for an example of a pathology report for prostate cancer.

There is also a study on Norwegian pathology reports for breast cancer, also from the Cancer Registry of Norway carried out by Weegar and Dalianis (2015). In total there were 40 pathology reports, of these 30 reports were used for developing a rule-based system and 10 reports for testing the system. An F-score of 0.86 was achieved. See Fig. 10.4 for an example of a pathology report for breast cancer written in Norwegian.

Generally, one conclusion is that most systems give around 80% precision and recall on average.

```
Biopsier fra venstre prostatalapp.
2: Prostatakarsinom, Gleason score 3+4=7(4/13 mm)
4: Prostatakarsinom, Gleason, score 3+3=6(0,5/12
mm)
1,3:Ikke påvist malignitet
Biopsier fra høyre prostatalapp:
5-7,9: HPIN og Prostatakarsinom, Gleason score
3+3=6(1/13 mm)
8: Prostatakarsinom, Gleason score 4+3=7(5/15,4/15
mm)
Perinevral infiltrasjon: ikke påvist
```

Translated to English:

```
Biopsies from the left lobe.
2: Prostate carcinoma, Gleason score 3+4=7(4/13 mm)
4: Prostate carcinoma, Gleason score 3+3=6(0.5/12
mm)
1,3:No signs of malignancy
Biopsies from the right lobe:
5-7,9: HPIN and adenocarcinoma, Gleason score
3+3=6(1/13 mm)
8: Prostate carcinoma, Gleason score 3+4=7(5/15 mm)
Perineural invasion: no signs
```

Fig. 10.3 A pseudonymised example of a Norwegian pathology report describing prostate biopsies. The text contains descriptions of 9 biopsies, four from the left side and five from the right side. Figure published in Weegar et al. (2017)

10.4.2 The Medical Text Extraction (Medtex) System

The Australian e-Health Research Centre (AeHRC) at CSIRO in Brisbane in Australia is closely connected with the Royal Brisbane and Women's Hospital. Nguyen et al. (2015) at the AeHRC constructed the Medical Text Extraction (Medtex) system, built in the Java programming language, which automatically processes a trickle feed of incoming pathology reports in HL7 format from the whole state of Queensland in Australia. The State of Queensland has almost 5 million inhabitants hence is almost as populated as Norway. Medtex uses NLP techniques, and the external resource of SNOMED CT for mapping and identifying medical concepts and abbreviations. A set of business rules was constructed for finding the structured data in the unstructured pathology text. The system was evaluated using a set of 220 unseen pathology reports and obtained an F-measure of 0.80 over seven categories.

In Fig. 10.5 we can see the interface of the CIPAR annotation system, which is part of the Medtex system.

```
Mammaresektat (ve. side) med infiltrerende duktalt
karsinom, histologisk grad 3
Tumordiameter 15 mm
Lavgradig DCIS med utstrekning 4 mm i kranial
retning fra tumor
Frie reseksjonsrender for infiltrerende tumor (3 mm
kranialt)
Lavgradig DCIS under 2 mm fra kraniale
reseksjonsrand

ER: ca 65 % av cellene positive
PGR: negativ
Ki-67: Hot-spot 23% positive celler. Cold spot 8%.
Gjennomsnitt 15%
HER-2: negativ
Tidl. BU 13:

3 sentinelle lymfeknuter uten påviste patologiske
forandringer
```

Translated to English:

```
Mamma specimen (le. side) with infiltrating ductal
carcinoma, histological grade 3
Tumor diameter 15 mm
Low-grade DCIS extending 4 mm in cranial direction
from the tumor
Free resection margins for infiltrating tumor (3 mm
cranially)
Low-grade DCIS less than 2 mm from the cranial
resection margin

ER: ca 65 % of the cells are positive
PGR: negative
Ki-67: Hot-spot 23% positive cells. Cold spot 8%.
Average 15%
HER-2: negative
Prev. BU 13:

3 sentinel lymph nodes without proven pathological
changes
```

Found concepts by a mockup system

```
Progesteronreseptorer (PGR): 1 (1 is a table value
that corresponds to "negative" in the text)
Samtidig Sentinell Node: 0
Østrogenreseptorer (ER): 4 (4 is a table value
that corresponds to "65 %" in the text)
KI67 Hotspot: 23
Tumors histologiske grad (Histological grade): 3
KI67 Gjennomsnitt hot/cold (Average): 15
Tumordiameter (Tumor diameter): 15
(In some cases the data is not found in the text
but in sketch attached to the pathology report).
```

Fig. 10.4 Extract from the free text part of an anonymised breast cancer pathology report in Norwegian (and its translation to English). This is a small subset of a report, with very few values, breasts cancer reports may have over 80 values. The data in the figure is made up and can not be linked to any individual (© 2015, Association for Computational Linguistics (ACL). All rights reserved. The Norwegian pathology text is reprinted with permission of ACL and the authors. Published in Weegar and Dalianis (2015). The translation to English and extracts from the free text are added in this publication)

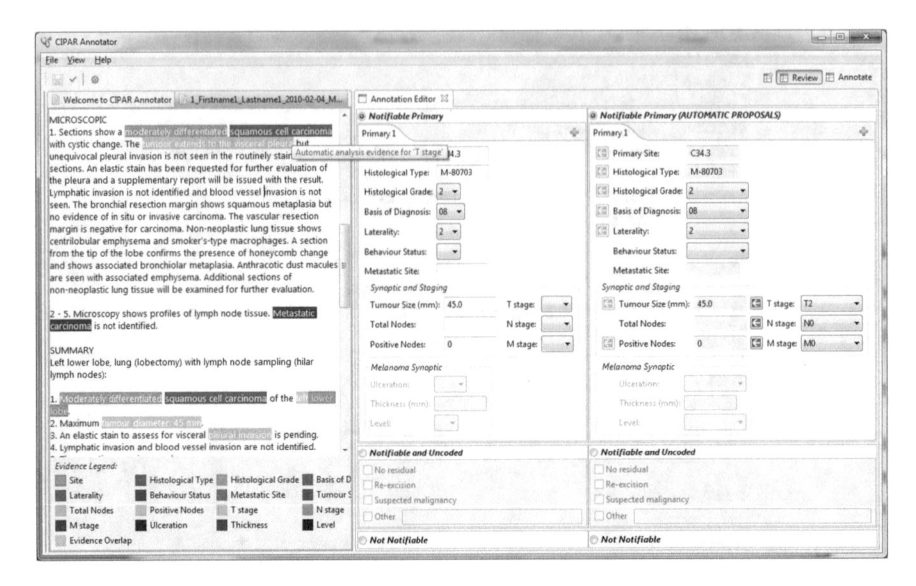

Fig. 10.5 Screenshot of the CIPAR annotation system. The Medtex software processes narrative reports and generates structured data to aid clinical staff in abstraction tasks, in this case lung cancer pathology reports. Taken from Figure 4 in Nguyen et al. (2015) (© 2015 Reprinted with permission from AMIA and the authors. Published in Nguyen et al. (2015))

10.5 Mining for Cancer Symptoms

There is a demand to predict diseases before they occur, or at least as early as possible, so the correct treatment can start early to minimise the suffering of the patient. One area in which to perform prediction is in the cancer domain. Cancer encompasses over 200 cancer types, where the name of the cancer type originates from the affected body organ. Each cancer type has its own and is treated according to each type.

Spasić et al. (2014) have written a nice review of different approaches for performing text mining for different cancer types. The conclusion is that most systems are based on pattern matching and rule-based methods for NER obtaining F-scores in the range of 0.80–0.90. To increase the performance, the systems need to deal with clinical sublanguage and non-standard abbreviations as well as misspellings and grammatical errors.

Jensen et al. (2012) focus on predicting the outcome for patients with a large number of diseases but also specifically in predicting the survival for breast cancer patients. Jensen et al. (2012) propose the use of multivariate models including variables such as age, sex, smoking etc. to make inferences on unknown data. Moreover, they recommend integrating patient record data with genetic data to understand genotype-phenotype relationships, but this requires careful consideration of ethical aspects.

In the domain of cancer text mining we can distinguish two aims and corresponding methods, one is the NER method, to find symptoms, disorders and affected body parts and the other is the classification of text to identify certain features which may indicate a type of cancer.

Weegar et al. (2015) carried out an approach to find symptoms of cervical cancer in Swedish patient records. Early detection of cervical cancer is crucial for the treatment and survival of the patient. The Clinical Entity Finder (CEF) was used, CEF is based on CRF++ and trained on records from Swedish internal medicine emergency units that are annotated for finding, disorder, body part and drug (Skeppstedt et al. 2014). The CEF was extended in the study with the rule-based NegEx negation detection system for Swedish by Weegar et al. (2015).

To evaluate the system two annotators who were also trained physicians, annotated a test set of patient records. The test data consisted of 646 records with patients diagnosed with cervical cancer that had been assigned the ICD-10 diagnosis code C53.

The inter-annotator agreement for finding, disorder and body part was on average an F-score of 0.677. The Clinical Entity Finder extended with NegEx obtained an average F-score of 0.667 (Weegar et al. 2015). The most frequent findings and disorders can be found in Table 10.3.

Zhao and Weng (2011) describe a system called iDiagnosis to predict pancreatic cancer. The system operates by combining PubMed knowledge and electronic health records (EHRs). iDiagnosis extracts 20 risk factors from PubMed abstracts. Keywords were used to classify the risk factors such as positive, negative or neutral associations. Risk factors can be in the classes of demographics, lifestyle, symptoms, co-morbidities and lab test results. Each variable of the model was assigned probabilities for patients with pancreatic cancer based on the information in PubMed, Prior probability for each variable was calculated using the EHRs. A model based on weighted Bayesian Network Inference (BNI) was trained, and pancreatic cancer could be predicted with the sensitivity (recall), specificity and accuracy of around 85%.

10.6 Text Summarisation and Translation of Patient Record

Automatic text summarisation is the technique where a computer program summarises a text. A text is entered into the computer and a summarised text is returned, which is a shorter non-redundant extract from the original text.

Text abstraction is when a completely new text abstract is created, this is similar to what a human does when a human reads the text, comprehends the text and then rephrases it into a completely new text with new word phrasing and new syntactical constructions—an abstract. To perform abstraction, the source text needs to be parsed syntactically and semantically into a formal representation, and then a completely new, shorter and non-redundant text is generated from the

Table 10.3 The most frequent findings, disorders and negations found in the physicians' notes

Most frequent findings and disorders	Nbr of instances	Most frequently negated findings and disorders	Nbr of negated instances	Findings and disorders with highest portion of negation	Portion negated
Cervixcancer (cervical cancer)	873	Besvär (trouble/problem)	338	Gynekologiska besvär (gynecological problems)	1.0
Besvär (trouble/problem)	790	Feber (fever)	243	Palpabla resistenser (palpable resistance)	1.0
Illamående (nausea)	677	Illamående (nausea)	198	Särskilda besvär (particular problems)	1.0
Mår bra (feels well)	662	Blödningar (bleedings)	171	Nytillkomna symtom (new symptoms)	0.96
Smärta (pain)	656	smärta (pain)	150	Nytillkomna besvär (new problems)	0.92
Tumör (tumor)	642	smärtor (pains)	126	Infektionstecken (signs of infection)	0.89
Smärter (pains)	629	Blödning (bleeding)	99	Biljud (murmur)	0.86
Feber (fever)	562	Infektionstecken (signs of infection)	91	Tumörstrukturer (tumour structures)	0.83
Cancer (cancer)	508	Tumör (tumor)	83	Tumörsuspekta förändringar (tumor suspicious changes)	0.82
Blödningar (bleedings)	491	Nytillkomna besvär (new troubles)	79	Subjektiva besvär (subjective problems)	0.8
Blödning (bleeding)	482	Buksmärtor (pain of the abdomen)	72	Tumörsuspekt (tumor suspicion)	0.80
Skivepitelcancer (squamous cell carcinoma)	428	Hydronefros (hydronephrosis)	65	Spridning (spreading)	0.78

Taken from Table 7 in Weegar et al. (2015) (© 2015 Reprinted with permission from AMIA and the authors. Published in Weegar et al. (2015))

formal representation, with new wording and syntactical structure but with the same meaning.

An automatic text summarisation system usually produces summary extracts, so-called extraction-based summarisation systems. An abstraction system is very difficult to construct therefore most systems are extraction based systems.

One of the first systems to create an automatic summary or abstract was described in Luhn (1958). The purpose was to create an informative extract to help researchers and scientist to cope with the growing number of publications. The extract was compiled from the most important parts of the article.

Later text summarisation systems were created to summarise new articles. Multi-document text summarisation systems have also been developed that analyse several similar news articles about the same topic to one non-redundant summary. Mani and Maybury (1999) have carried out a compilation of the state of the art in text summarisation including an historical review.

An extractive text summarisation system works basically by splitting a text into sentences and then finding the most information intensive or meaning bearing words of the texts. The meaning bearing parts are usually title words, initial sentences (especially in news text) and sentences containing named entities, such as personal names, organisations, locations and numerical values, but also sentences containing verbs that are frequent. Stop words, which are not meaning bearing words, are filtered away.

All these measurement points are put together to give each sentence a numerical ranking or scoring. The ranking is in turn normalised depending on the length of the sentence, since longer sentences tend to contain more information than shorter sentences. Finally, the summary is compiled from the highest ranking sentences in consecutive order. The length of the summary is decided beforehand or by a cut-off value. The final summary is shorter, hopefully coherent and almost as information intensive as the original text.

There are many different ways to perform automatic text summarisation, the example just described is a rule-based or heuristic (rule of thumb) approach, but there are also approaches that use statistics from large corpora or pure machine learning methods trained on example texts and their corresponding abstracts. The algorithms based on these methods can then produce a summary that is similar to other learned summaries or abstracts.

There is also a method called query based or keyword based text summarisation that customises the summary around what the user wants to read about. The summary is then focused around the specific keywords the user enters to the system. This approach is slightly similar to the text snippets focused around the search words in the ranked search list obtained when carrying out a regular search in a search engine.

There is a group of text summarisation systems using distributional semantics and word embeddings to construct summaries see Hassel (2007), Hassel and Sjöbergh (2006) and specifically for clinical text by Moen et al. (2016) that will be discussed in the next section.

10.6.1 Summarising the Patient Record

One requirement from the physicians regarding summarisation of patient records is to summarise the whole healthcare episodes or period of patient treatment into a discharge summary, until today there have been few approaches.

Early work on understanding the content of the patient records is described in LifeLines where information is extracted and presented in a timeline (Plaisant et al. 1998), this is described in Sect. 3.3 and specifically in Fig. 3.2.

Pivovarov and Elhadad (2015) review different approaches of summarising a patient record, but none of them really address the challenge of creating a discharge summary from a healthcare episode.

Van Vleck and Elhadad (2010) describe an approach to find the most relevant information in the form of clinical problems to be included in a patient summary. The authors treat this problem as a classification problem. The classifier is trained on a corpus of patient notes and their corresponding problem list using the two machine learning algorithms Naïve-Bayes and J48 (C4.5) implemented in the Weka toolkit. One issue was how to exclude negated events, or events in the summary that had not occurred yet. The classifiers obtained an accuracy of 82% and an F-score of 0.62 on this task.

Aramaki et al. (2009) propose a text-summarising system TEXT2TABLE, which extracts relevant information from the patient record and presents it in a table. The problem is similar to the one in Van Vleck and Elhadad (2010) to filter out non-relevant information from the patient records as negated events, or events that will happen in the future or may happen. The authors trained their algorithms on 435 Japanese discharge summaries in which seven different events types that should be *excluded* in the summary, such as *negation, future, (planned) purpose, S/O (suspected disease), necessity, intend, possible, recommend* (by other doctor) and their modalities were annotated. The SVM classifier was trained to decide whether an event had actually occurred or not. The experimental results obtained an F-score of 0.858.

Liu (2009) used the MEAD text summarisation system made for English text to summarise Finnish nursing narratives. The author adapted the system to Finnish. In total 252 text summaries were created and evaluated; however, no evaluation results are presented.

Moen et al. (2016) did excellent work in comparing a number of summarisation methods to create a discharge summary from a consecutive number of documents for an individual patient. 66,884 care episodes in Finnish were used describing patients with cardiac problems. The constructed automatic summarisation system was an extraction-based, multi-document summarisation system since each patient record contain multiple documents used as inputs to the text summariser. The summarisation system used distributional semantics and specifically the random indexing method, to create a word space model for extracting features for the different summarisation methods used.

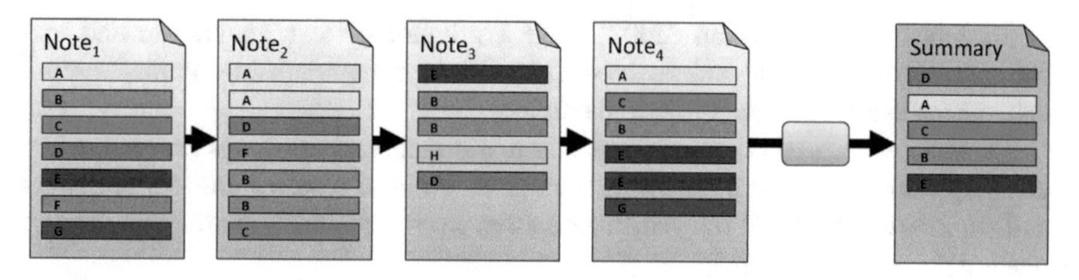

Fig. 10.6 Example of automatic discharge summary creation. Redundant information is removed and high scoring information is added to the beginning of the summary from highest to lowest, low scoring information G, F and H, is excluded. Taken from Figure 3 in Moen et al. (2016), licensed under Creative Commons

Sentences from each document in the care episode are extracted and composed into the automatic discharge summary, see Fig. 10.6.

The authors compare eight different summarisation methods. The summariser uses sentence topic clustering and topic scoring to score the sentences. Topic clustering was used specifically to obtain redundancy reduction. Redundancy can occur both within one document but also across over several documents that are going to be summarised. The similarity measurement for sentence similarity is based on distributional semantics.

One of the best performing summarisation methods was the composite method that combines parts from other methods such as sentence ranking and normalisation of sentence length, the top high ranking sentences are selected for the final summary.

During the experiment each care episode was summarised using eight different summarisation methods producing in total eight different discharge summaries (where one of the "methods" was an original human-made discharge summary). Three domain experts evaluated the discharge summaries produced. In addition, four different evaluation metrics from the ROUGE[12] evaluation package were used. In total 156 care episodes were utilised for the automatic evaluation. This work was also part of Moen's PhD thesis, see Moen (2016).

10.6.2 *Other Approaches in Summarising the Patient Record*

There are also approaches using *natural language generation (NLG)* techniques to transfer information directly from structured data to text. Portet et al. (2009) used data from a neonatal intensive care data department to create a flow text description of how the baby feels directed towards the parents and relatives.

[12]ROUGE score is a metric that uses unigram co-occurrences between summary pairs: the machine produced one and the gold standard or human produced abstract to calculate the quality of the summary (or machine translation). https://en.wikipedia.org/wiki/ROUGE_(metric). Accessed 2018-01-11.

Torgersson and Falkman (2002) used a mixture of text generation and text summarisation to create an easily navigated and comprehensible patient record called MedView in the area of oral medicine.

Elhadad et al. (2005) present an automatic summarisation system where the discharge summary of the patient is used as an input to search PubMed, to extract and summarise the most relevant information for the patient's characteristics into one article.

Johnson et al. (2008) used a similar approach but took the textual input from the physician, together with other structured information from the patient record, to structure the patient records and create a summary.

10.6.3 Summarising Medical Scientific Text

Sarker et al. (2013) studied an approach to summarise query-focused information from medical scientific text. The text originate from the *Journal of Family Practice* that is aimed at general practitioners. The corpus studied contains almost three thousand medical scientific articles document, of which 1319 were set aside for evaluation, the rest were used for training. The abstracts of the documents are structured and only these are used for training and evaluation. Each document is associated with a clinical query.

Both the query and the content of the document was used to create a summary. Eleven different algorithms were tested, of which five were baseline algorithms (see Sect. 6.3 for the explanation of baseline) and the rest were machine learning algorithms trained on the training corpus. The QSpec (grid search) summarisation algorithm gave the best results using standard sentence scoring rules for text summarisation (each part of the sentence contributes to the total scoring), but where the weights for each sentence score were optimised using grid search. The QSpec system obtained a percentile rank of 96.8% outperforming all the other systems tested in the study.

10.6.4 Simplification of the Patient Record for Laypeople

Related to the summarisation of the patient record is the simplification of the patient record for the layreader. This function has become relevant as individual patient records have become accessible on the Internet for the patients in many countries. The patient can hence read his or hers patient record on-line; however, the patient record is difficult to understand for laypeople since it contains many specialised medical terms and also very domain specific language (Ramesh et al. 2013).

Ramesh et al. (2013) have shown that their system Clinical Notes Aid (NoteAid) improved comprehension of the patient record among laypeople. NoteAid translates the medical jargon in the patient record to a consumer-oriented lay language, it uses

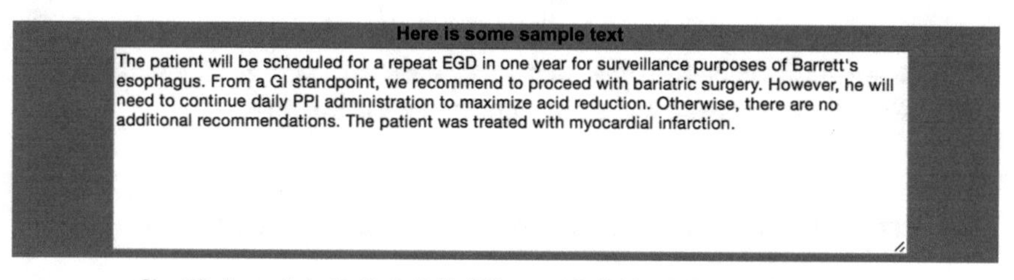

Fig. 10.7 Screenshot of Clinical Notes Aid showing a clinical text where a medical concept is explained in a pop up menu. From the online demo, http://www.clinicalnotesaid.org/emrreadability/notesaid.uwm. Accessed 2018-01-11

Wikipedia, MedlinePlus (a disease dictionary) and UMLS to support the creation of the simplified text. Progress notes are considered to be more difficult to comprehend for laypeople. NoteAid improved comprehensibility most for progress notes using Wikipedia as a dictionary, the results were also statistically significant. See Fig. 10.7 for a screenshot of NoteAid.

Kandula et al. (2010) performed an approach to simplify medical patient record text in English. Texts containing long sentences and difficult words are considered to be hard to read. The authors used a part of speech tagger and a grammar simplifier to replace sentences longer that 10 words with two or more shorter sentences and semantically difficult terms with easier synonyms. The evaluation used the *cloze test* where every fifth word was replaced with a blank and the reviewers were asked to fill in the missing term. The easier it is to replace the missing term, the easier the text is to read. A cloze test on the patient records showed a statistically significant improvement for the simplified patient records from 35.8% to 43.6% in cloze score.

For Swedish there has been one approach for lexical simplification of clinical text with the aim of making it more comprehensible for laypeople. The approach was to resolve unknown words as compounds words, abbreviations or misspellings (Grigonyte et al. 2014). The method used was to first detect and expand all abbreviations, the remaining words may be compounds, unknown words or misspelled words. Finally unknown words are resolved as either as compounded known words, abbreviations or misspellings. The results obtained were: 91.1% precision for abbreviations, 83.5% precision for compound splitting and finally 83.9% precision for spelling corrections.

For Swedish a ground breaking study on grammatical simplification of news text was carried out by Anna Decker in her master's thesis (Decker 2003). She proposed 25 formalised simplification rules. Decker used newspaper articles written in Swedish for immigrants, and compared parallel text, both original and simplified, to find patterns and create her simplification rules. The simplification rules for Swedish are implemented in the web service SCREAM[13] by Falkenjack et al. (2017). SCREAM also contains a text summariser for Swedish.

10.7 ICD-10 Diagnosis Code Assignment and Validation

There are around 32,000 different ICD-10 diagnosis codes that are used for classifying diseases. The coding is mainly carried out for statistical, administrative and financial reasons but is also useful for the physician to quickly perceive what codes diseases, the patient record is assigned with. The coding is performed by the treating physician but also by specific trained coders. The ICD-10 code is assigned to the discharge letter of the patient.

It is important to have correct and reliable statistics when planning healthcare. However, in an investigation carried out by National Board of Health and Welfare in Sweden (Socialstyrelsen), 4200 patient records were reviewed and it was found that there were 20% errors in the ICD-10 codes. In another investigation encompassing 1.5 million patient records, the National Board found that 1.2% of the main diagnoses were missing (Socialstyrelsen 2010).

Because of these challenges it would be valuable to have a system that automatically assigns ICD-10 diagnosis codes to a discharge summary, or at least proposes probable codes to the treating physician or coder. It would also be valuable to have a system that validates the manually assigned codes and warns when something is wrong.

In 2007 there was a shared task to automatically assign ICD-9 codes to radiology reports. The shared task was called the *Computational Medicine Center's 2007 Medical Natural Language Processing Challenge*. Their data consisted of a training and development set of 978 documents and a test set of 976 documents in the radiology domain. The records were assigned with 45 different ICD-9 labels in the form of 780.6, 786.2 etc, which in this example refer to fever and cough, Pestian et al. (2007).

Over 44 teams participated in the shared task, most approaches used rule-based methods; the second best team consist of Farkas and Szarvas (2008), that used a combined rule-based and machine learning approach (the Maximum Entropy classifier) and obtained an F-score of 0.903 on the training set and an F-score of 0.889 on the test.

Perotte et al. (2014) extended the approach using 22,815 non-empty discharge summaries from the MIMIC II database of which 90%, or 20,533 documents, were used for training and 10%, or 2282 document, were used for evaluation. In total 5030 ICD-9 codes were assigned to the documents, some documents were, of course, assigned multiple codes. The best results for the machine learning approach were

[13]SCREAM Textförenklare (in Swedish), http://www.ida.liu.se/projects/scream/webapp/. Accessed 2018-01-11.

obtained using a hierarchy-based SVM classifier that gave an F-score of 0.40. It assigned an average 6.31 codes per document.

Suominen et al. (2008) used both the Regularized Least Squares (RLS) classifier that is closely related to SVM and the RIPPER rule induction-based learning method. The RIPPER rule induction-based learning method was the best of the two methods and obtained an F-score of 0.877 giving the team a third place in the challenge.

Studies for automatic ICD-10 code assignment for French, Bulgarian, Danish, Swedish and Japanese respectively have been carried out by Lavergne et al. (2016), Boytcheva (2011), Roque et al. (2011a), Henriksson and Hassel (2013) and Aramaki et al. (2014).

Kavuluru et al. (2015) experimented with 93,694 French death certificates and assigned 377,677 ICD-10 codes (3457 unique codes). The data was used for a shared task where the best team obtained an F-score of 0.848.

In Fig. 10.8 we can see the results of building a word space model from 408,144 Swedish annotated patient records and their corresponding 35,185 ICD-10 diagnosis codes using the Random Forest algorithm. The data originate from the Stockholm EPR Corpus's first 5 months of year 2008. This constructed word space model can be used both to find which ICD-10 code corresponds best with a certain word, and which medical term or symptom corresponds best with a certain ICD-10 code.

In Henriksson et al. (2011) the random indexing experiments showed that of the top 10 generated candidates, 20% were correct and 77% were partially correct. The approach was refined in Henriksson and Hassel (2013) where the dimensionality was increased and gave up to 18% better results.

Stanfill et al. (2010) have written an overview of ICD-8, ICD-9 and ICD-10 automatic coding of patient records; almost a historical review is carried out. The best performing systems obtained F-scores of around 0.90 for ICD-9 codes.

Hosta (cough)

J18.9 - Pneumoni, ospecificerad (Pneumonia, unspecified)
J15.9 - Bakteriell pneumoni, ospecificerad (Bacterial pneumonia, unspecified)
H66.9 - Mellanöreinflammation, ej specificerad som varig / icke varig (Otitis media, unspecified)
J20.9 - Akut bronkit, ospecificerad, (Acute bronchitis, unspecified)
B34.9 - Virusinfektion, ospecificerad, (Viral infection, unspecified)
G96.9 - Sjukdom i centrala nervsystemet, ospecificerad (Disorder of central nervous system, unspecified)
I50.9 - Hjärtinsufficiens, ospecificerad (Heart failure, unspecified)
F48.9 - Neurotiskt syndrom, ospecificerat (Neurotic disorder, unspecified)
C34.9 - Icke specificerad lokalisation av malign tumör i bronk & lunga (Bronchus or lung, unspecified)
L64.9 - Androgen alopeci, ospecificerad (Androgenic alopecia, unspecified)

Fig. 10.8 Example of ICD-10 code suggestions (© 2009 The authors—reprinted with permission from the authors. Published in Dalianis et al. (2009))

Koopman et al. (2015a) experimented with death certificates from New South Wales in Australia to classify diabetes, influenza, pneumonia and HIV. A set of 340,142 death certificates was divided into 80% for training and 20% for a test set. All death certificates were coded with ICD-10 diagnosis codes. Both the machine learning-based method SVM (from the Weka toolkit) and a rule-based method based on keyword-matching rules were used. The keywords were selected with assistance from domain experts on words that characterise each disease. Both methods yielded very similar results with an F-score of around 0.96.

10.7.1 Natural Language Generation from SNOMED CT

SNOMED CT is a very complex hierarchical medical terminology that contains many separate pieces of information with the aim of describing a disorder, its cause, symptoms and in which body part the disorder occurs. The concepts are coded in SNOMED CT and are difficult for a human to validate. See for example the IHTSDO SNOMED CT Browser and its description of scarlet fever in Fig. 10.9,

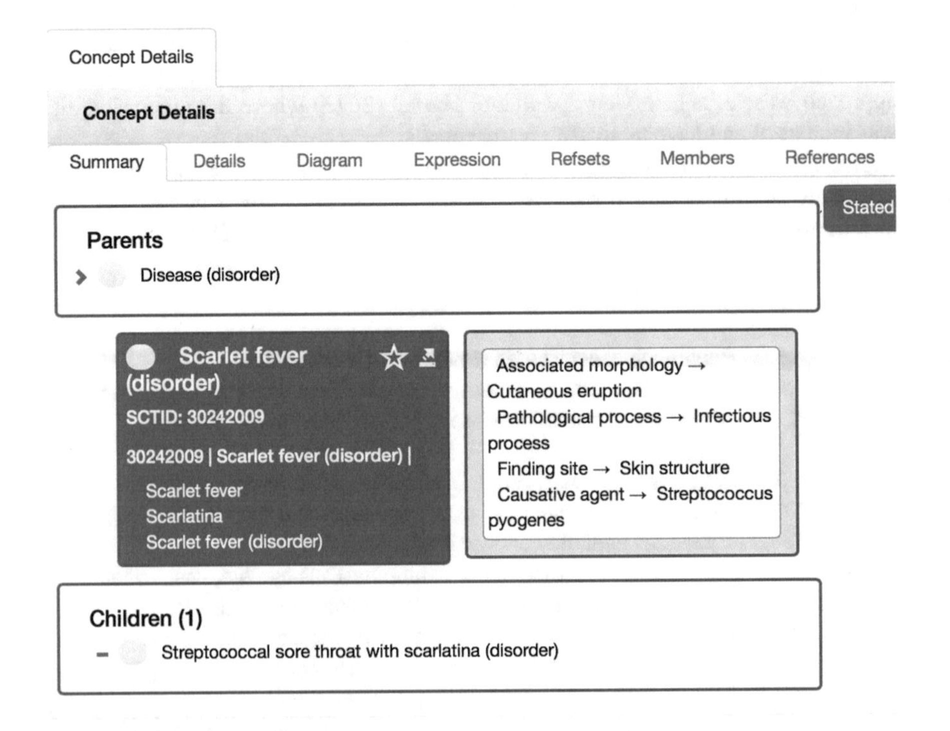

Fig. 10.9 The IHTSDO SNOMED CT Browser and its description of scarlet fever, the browser is described in Sect. 5.2

> ***Input:*** *Scharlakansfeber*
> ***Output:*** *Scharlakansfeber är en eruption och hudsjukdom orsakad av streptokocker. Orsaken till sjukdomen är Streptococcus pyogenes. Sjukdomen finns i hud och hudstruktur och hud.*
> ***(Translated with Google translate to English:***
> ***Input:*** *Scarlet fever*
> ***Output:*** *Scarlet fever is an eruption and skin disease caused by streptococci. The cause of the disease is Streptococcus pyogenes. The disease is found in skin and skin structure and skin.*

Fig. 10.10 Example of natural language output from the SNOgen system, when entering the disorder *scharlakansfeber* (in Eng: scarlet fever) in SNOMED CT format and obtaining the Swedish natural language text output. Below is the corresponding machine translated English text (© 2014 The authors—reprinted with permission from the authors. Published in Kanhov (2014))

therefore, an approach to automatically generate natural language text from the SNOMED CT structure has been carried out using a prototype called SNOGEN.

The same example describing scarlet fever in SNOMED CT format is entered into the SNOGEN natural language generator. The generated natural language text describes a certain part of the disorder in the context of the cause and where in the body it occurs. The natural language discourse makes it easier to understand and validate the description of scarlet fever expressed in SNOMED CT format, see Fig. 10.10 for an example of *natural language generation* text of Scarlet fever from SNOMED CT (Kanhov et al. 2012; Kanhov 2014).

10.8 Search Cohort Selection and Similar Patient Cases

10.8.1 Comorbidities

Comorbidity means a disorder co-occurs with other disorders as well as a disorder that may cause other disorders. If a patient obtains one disorder which other disorder or disorders are expected to occur sequentially? One application for detecting this is the visualisation tool Comorbidity-View[14] available on the Internet. Comorbidity-View is applied on part of the HEALTH BANK data, more exactly on all patient records from the Karolinska University Hospital encompassing the years 2006–2008, in total 605,587 patients; and visualises them in the form of ICD-10 codes and patients in a comorbidity network, see Fig. 10.11.

The Comorbidity-View tool is a useful tool for quickly exploring the available patient record data, in terms of patients, gender, ages and ICD-10 codes; however, one drawback is that it does not have temporal information on which disorder

[14]Comorbidity-View, https://www2.dsv.su.se/comorbidityview-demo/. Accessed 2018-01-11.

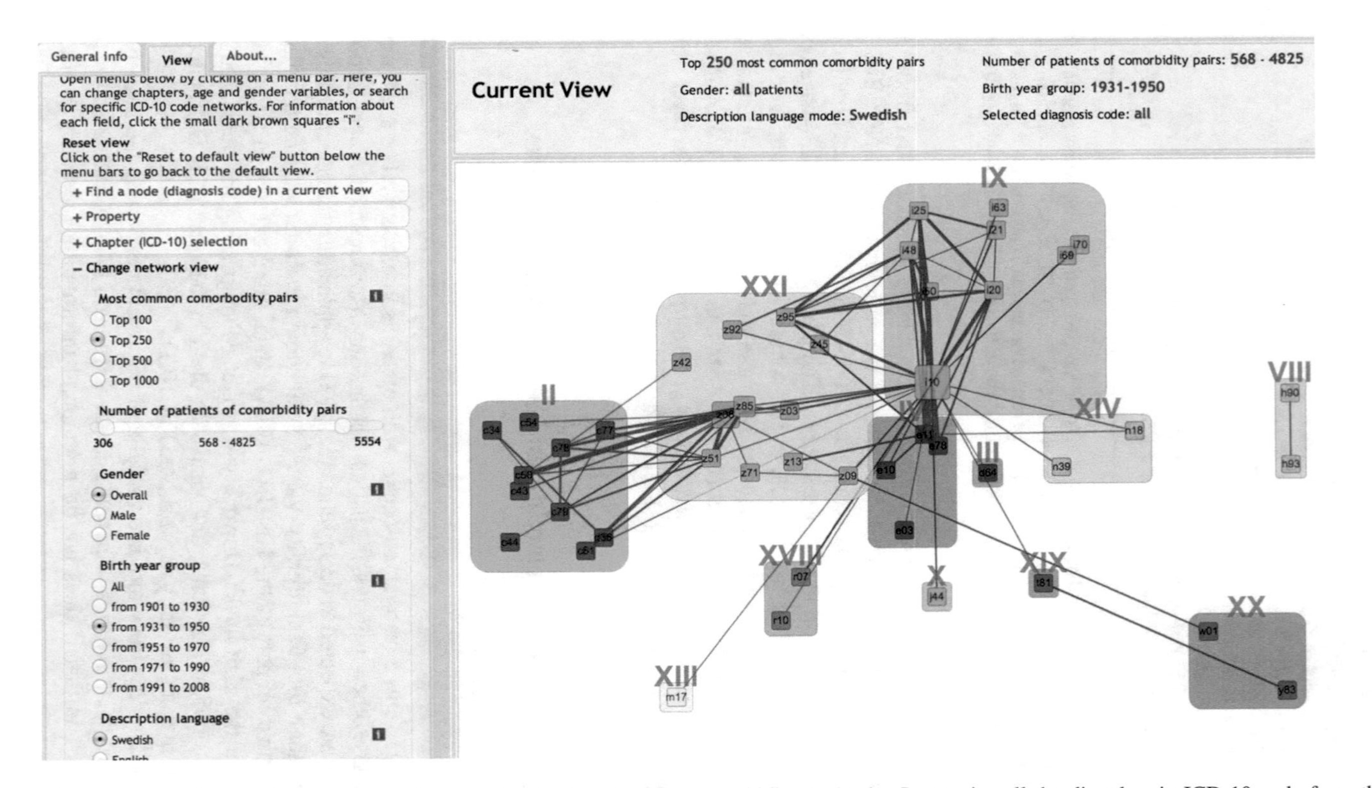

Fig. 10.11 Screenshot of Comorbidity-View, which is a visualisation tool for comorbidity networks. It contains all the disorders in ICD-10 code form that patient records have been assigned. The data contains 605,587 patients over the years 2006–2008 from the Karolinska University Hospital. The thicker the line in Comorbidity-View the more patients who had both ICD-10 codes. The boxes correspond to chapters of ICD-10 codes (Tanushi et al. 2011)

occurred first, second etc. In Comorbidity-View all disorder pairs are presented in the same temporal order.

One similar approach to detect comorbidities using text mining is presented by Roque et al. (2011b), involving Danish clinical corpus containing 5543 psychiatric patients records, their disorders and corresponding manually assigned ICD-10 diagnosis codes.

The methods used for automatically detecting ICD-10 codes were purely rule-based using lists of words from ICD-10 dictionaries, negation detection or detection of relatives of the patient.

31,662 ICD-10 codes were automatically extracted, of which 22,956 were disqualified since they either were negated or they were connected to a relative of the patient. Manual evaluation was carried out on 48 patients and a precision of 87.78% was calculated, the value of the recall is not mentioned.

The most frequent ICD-10 chapter using the manually assigned ICD-10 codes was chapter V *Mental and behavioral disorders* After text mining for other disorders and automatic assignment of ICD-10 diagnosis codes, chapter X *Diseases of the respiratory system* and chapter XIX *Injury, poisoning and certain other consequences of external causes* were more common. The comorbidity network grew significantly after the text mining and this shows that psychiatric patients often have other disorders that are not recorded in their patient record.

10.8.2 Information Retrieval from Electronic Patient Records

A number of shared tasks within clinical text mining have been carried out, for example the TREC 2013 Medical Record Track as well as the ShARe/CLEF eHealth Evaluation Lab from 2013 up to 2016. All shared tasks used electronic patient records that had been de-identified and pseudonymised. All participating teams in the shared task needed to sign confidentiality agreements due to the possible sensitivity of the patient records.

In TREC 2013, the tasks were similar to the previous Text REtrieval Conferences (TREC) using patient records as document collections. The task was constructed in the domain of *cohort* studies, to find a group of patients sharing similar properties. This was simulated by retrieving a particular topic from 50 selected topics contained in 17,264 electronic patient records in English. Each record corresponds to a patient. The records were annotated with ICD-9 diagnosis codes,[15] which also could be used to retrieve topics. Voorhees and Hersh (2012) also reported the challenge of classifying negated findings and negated disorders, which is specific to this type of text.

ShARe/CLEF eHealth Evaluation 2013 contained three different tasks using clinical text written in English (Suominen et al. 2013):

- The first task was to identify and normalise disorders and map them to SNOMED CT.

[15]ICD-9 diagnosis codes are used in the US, and are an earlier revision of ICD-10.

- The second task was to expand abbreviations and acronyms.
- The third task was a traditional Q&A task for patients, but using clinical reports that the patient may ask questions about.

10.8.3 Search Engine Solr

There is one useful and well-known search engine for indexing and retrieving documents, and (of course) electronic patient records, called Solr,[16] previously Lucene. Solr has, for example, been used in the study by Korkontzelos et al. (2012) regarding clinical trials but also in the shared task within precision medicine described in Roberts et al. (2016). The official name of the shared task in precision medicine was *TREC 2014 Clinical Decision Support Track*. Precision medicine means customised treatment to each individual patient. The task to use patient cases, described in free text, as queries to find the best treatment for the patient among 733,138 scientific articles in Pubmed Central (PMC). Pubmed is an online digital database of freely available full-text biomedical literature.

10.8.4 Supporting the Clinician in an Emergency Department with the Radiology Report

One problem with radiology reports in emergency departments is the time delay between the report from the radiologist and the clinical treatment of the patient. The first radiology report might miss limb fractures and the patient is sent home, after review of the X-rays the radiologist might discover limb fractures and the patient is then re-admitted for treatment. In an study carried by Koopman et al. (2015b) the authors used machine learning techniques to solve this problem.

2378 freetext radiology reports on limb structures from three large Australian public hospitals were studied. The reports are very short, an average only 47 words. Radiologists carried out a review of these free-text radiology reports and classified them as normal or abnormal, i.e. with some fracture on the limb. The machine learning system based on SVM in the Weka toolkit was trained on these classified radiology reports and obtained an F-score of 0.92. This gives the opportunity for the radiologist to only review 11% of the original 2378 radiology reports and to considerably diminish the time delay.

In a nice demonstrator called RadSearch, Bevan Koopman demonstrates the ability to search radiology reports and simultaneously obtain cohorts of patients with a certain medical condition, see Fig. 10.12.

---

[16]Solr, http://lucene.apache.org/solr/. Accessed 2018-01-11.

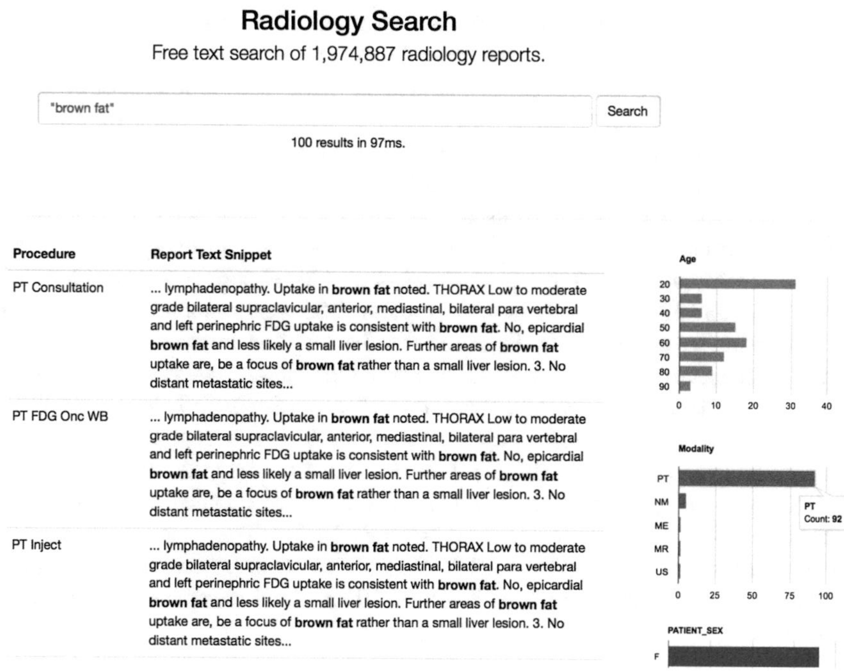

Radiology Search

Free text search of 1,974,887 radiology reports.

"brown fat" Search

100 results in 97ms.

Procedure	Report Text Snippet
PT Consultation	... lymphadenopathy. Uptake in **brown fat** noted. THORAX Low to moderate grade bilateral supraclavicular, anterior, mediastinal, bilateral para vertebral and left perinephric FDG uptake is consistent with **brown fat**. No, epicardial **brown fat** and less likely a small liver lesion. Further areas of **brown fat** uptake are, be a focus of **brown fat** rather than a small liver lesion. 3. No distant metastatic sites...
PT FDG Onc WB	... lymphadenopathy. Uptake in **brown fat** noted. THORAX Low to moderate grade bilateral supraclavicular, anterior, mediastinal, bilateral para vertebral and left perinephric FDG uptake is consistent with **brown fat**. No, epicardial **brown fat** and less likely a small liver lesion. Further areas of **brown fat** uptake are, be a focus of **brown fat** rather than a small liver lesion. 3. No distant metastatic sites...
PT Inject	... lymphadenopathy. Uptake in **brown fat** noted. THORAX Low to moderate grade bilateral supraclavicular, anterior, mediastinal, bilateral para vertebral and left perinephric FDG uptake is consistent with **brown fat**. No, epicardial **brown fat** and less likely a small liver lesion. Further areas of **brown fat** uptake are, be a focus of **brown fat** rather than a small liver lesion. 3. No distant metastatic sites...

Age
20
30
40
50
60
70
80
90
0 10 20 30 40

Modality
PT
NM
ME
MR
US
PT Count: 92
0 25 50 75 100

PATIENT_SEX
F

Fig. 10.12 Screenshot of Radsearch, a tool for extracting cohorts of patients with a certain medical condition in radiology. In this case the search terms are *brown fat* (The screenshot is a courtesy of Bevan Koopman)

10.8.5 Incident Reporting

Incident reporting has been mentioned previously, for example to detect healthcare associated infections, see Sect. 10.1, and adverse drug event detection, see Sect. 10.2, but there are some other types of incident reporting, for example to detect adverse events such as pressure sores, patient falls, device failures, nutrition problems, surgical complications as well as healthcare associated infections.

One way of detecting adverse events is to use the *Global Trigger Tool (GTT)* the method which is a manual method to review patient records for trigger words. According to the method there are different groups of adverse events, and within each group specific adverse events that one should review the records for. Doupi et al. (2015) describe one approach at the Karolinska University Hospital in Stockholm, Sweden, where the method was implemented as a semi-automatic method to find candidates for manual review by clinical personnel. The method is called *Modifierad Automatiserad (Modified Automatised) GTT, (MAG)*. MAG searches for triggers both in the structured information and in the free text of the patient record. The results are then reviewed and summarised by the tool. The system was developed in SAS Institute software.

For an academic article see Gerdes and Hardahl (2012) for an approach using SAS® Text Miner and SAS® Enterprise Content Categorization to find pressure ulcers (pressure injuries) in Danish patient records. The approach obtained a negative predictive value, i.e. a value for not finding indications of pressure ulcers was 97%, which is very good, but the positive predictive value for finding indications of pressure ulcers was only 56%, which is comparatively low.

In Australia an approach is used to classify incident reports into types of incidents. Around 10% of all admissions to acute care hospitals result in an adverse event and an incident report. Wang et al. (2017) performed the following study: from 137,522 submitted incident reports 6000 were randomly selected and in turn manually annotated by three experts. Part of this set was divided into a balanced subset of the following 11 incident types *falls, medications, pressure injury, aggression, documentation,*[17] *blood product, patient identification, infection, clinical handover, deteriorating patient* and *others*. This subset comprised in total 260 reports in each class in total 2860 reports, using the Support Vector Machine (SVM) algorithm gave an F-score of 0.783. Another imbalanced dataset of 5950 reports was also annotated and gave an F-score of 0.739. The inter-rater reliability for determining incident types was 0.93 Cohen's κ calculated on a small separate training set for the tree annotators. See Sect. 10.2.4 about adverse event detection systems.

10.8.6 Hypothesis Generation

One more domain is the generation and testing of new hypotheses. One example of this is presented in Dalianis et al. (2009), where the document clustering system Infomat[18] based on the vector space model was used. 4000 electronic patient records in Swedish from geriatric clinics were extracted from the Stockholm EPR corpus. The free text fields *bedömning* (assessment) and the structured entry gender were used for the clustering experiments. 62% of the patients in the corpus were women and 38% were men. One observation was that more documents describing female patients contained the words (translated from Swedish) *crutch, pelvis, femur, walkers, support, lift* and *broken bone*, than documents describing male patients, one new hypothesis is therefore that more women than men suffer from bone brittleness. There were also more men than women who had problems with memory and dementia. The hypothesis that more women than men suffers from bone brittleness was also supported after some preliminary literature studies. Figure 10.13 shows a screenshot of Infomat applied on electronic patient records in geriatrics. The "bone brittleness" words in Swedish can been seen in the middle of the figure in the boxes and these are also gathered in the diagonal line of the Infomat tool.

[17] The type "documentation", include various errors in documentation, that lead to an incident.

[18] Informat, http://www.csc.kth.se/tcs/projects/infomat/infomat/. Accessed 2018-01-11.

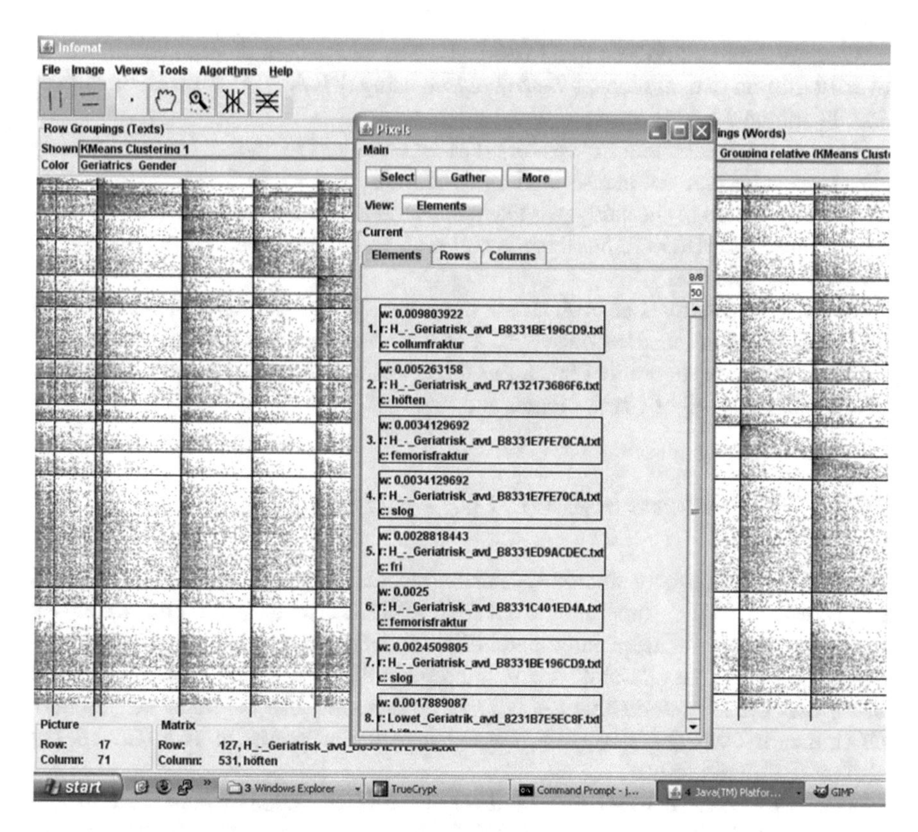

Fig. 10.13 Screenshot of hypothesis generation in geriatrics using the Infomat clustering tool. The "bone brittleness" words in Swedish such as *collumfractur, femorisfracture, höft (hip) etc.* indicating female patients can be observed in the boxes

10.8.7 Practical Use of SNOMED CT

Regarding SNOMED CT, there are two studies describing the use of the terminology (Lee et al. 2013, 2014). The first study (Lee et al. 2013) is an interview survey and the other study (Lee et al. 2014) is a literature review.

In the first study (Lee et al. 2013), called "A survey of SNOMED CT implementations", the authors contacted over 50 users of SNOMED CT in February 2012, this resulted in 14 interviews for 13 different implementation in over eight countries. The interviewees were professionals ranging from physicians, academics, clinical terminologists and software developers to vendors.

Some of the success factors for the use of SNOMED CT were: simplicity, involvement by clinicians and ease of demonstrating value and training.

The most common success factor was keeping the user interface simple for clinicians, hiding the complexity of SNOMED CT.

One implementation was in a historical electronic patient record system, where over 10 million patient records were analysed using SNOMED CT resulting in over 20,000 unique descriptions.

One other implementation was for assisting clinicians in finding new useful body site terms to be used for measuring blood pressure.

The conclusion of the study was that a lot effort and resources have been spent on developing SNOMED CT but there is still much work required to bring SNOMED CT into practical use.

In the second study (Lee et al. 2014), the authors investigated over 488 articles on SNOMED CT published between 2001 and 2012. Most articles comprised academic work mostly on a theoretical level, but there was also work on how to harmonise SNOMED CT to other terminologies and standards.

10.8.8 ICD-10 and SNOMED CT Code Mapping

There have been many attempts, mostly manual, to map from either ICD-10 to SNOMED CT or sometimes from SNOMED CT to ICD-10. The reason for the mapping is to achieve interoperability between the terminologies, or at least some degree of interoperability. The interoperability will make it possible to use SNOMED CT in systems that use ICD-10 coding, and also the other way around. Of course SNOMED CT is much more expressful and powerful than ICD-10, but also more difficult to use.

One early method was carried out by Wang et al. (2008) where their system mapped ICPC-2 PLUS to SNOMED CT with a precision of 96.46% and overall recall of 44.89%.

The mapping was performed both as string mapping including substring matching after removing stop words etc, and expanding abbreviation matching, but also mapping using WordNet synonym lexicon matching (in English), UMLS mapping, and finally post-coordination mapping, where several terms in a concept were extracted and matched partially into a SNOMED CT procedure.

ICPC-2 PLUS (also known as the BEACH coding system) is a coding system developed for primary care in Australia. It contains 7410 concepts. Wang et al. (2008) used only 5971 of these concepts to map to SNOMED CT that contains over 300,000 concepts.

Andersson and Sjöberg (2016) carried out a master's thesis work where they mapped the Swedish version of SNOMED CT to the Swedish version of ICD-10 using lexical similarity. The normalisation of the text descriptions included non-functional word (stop word) removal, stemming and decompounding using a specially built decompounder for Swedish medical words.

Andersson and Sjöberg (2016) constructed different matching algorithms including semantic similarity for SNOMED CT and ICD-10, meaning that if two concepts describe the same thing they are semantically similar. 948 ICD-10 concepts in the test set were evaluated by 10 domain experts obtaining a precision of 68.6% and a recall of 69.9%.

10.8.9 Analysing the Patient's Speech

Dementia is a gradual decline of cognitive abilities, often resulting from neurodegeneration. To detect early signs of dementia one project was carried out analysing the patient's speech. The patient's speech is recognised by a speech recogniser and then converted to text that is analysed with natural language processing methods.

In a study by Fraser et al. (2015) the DementiaBank corpus was used, which contains 167 patients diagnosed with "possible" or "probable" Alzheimer's disease. The DementiaBank corpus contains 240 narrative samples, and 97 controls sample provide another 233 speech samples. A method based on linguistic features was applied both to the pure speech and to the recognised speech in the form of text. The annotated data was used to train machine learning classifiers, such as logistic regression (LR) and support vector machines (SVM), to automatically classify patients with Alzheimer's disease and healthy patients. The approach gave an accuracy of over 81%.

The results from the research of Fraser et al. (2015) are currently being transferred into a Swedish context and adapted to Swedish dementia patients. The Swedish study will extend the speech analysis with eye movement analysis of the patients and other cognitive markers. The planned work is described in Kokkinakis et al. (2017).

10.8.10 MYCIN and Clinical Decision Support

There is a research area called clinical decision systems, these systems support the physician in his or her decision on diagnosis and treatment. The area has it origins in the expert systems and knowledge based systems of the 1980s. There has been discussion on the ethics on such systems, that is if they give the wrong decision to the physician, who is the responsible the machine or the physician?

One well-known clinical decision system is MYCIN, developed in 1970s, for detecting and giving treatment advice on blood diseases such as bacteremia and meningitis. It contained over 600 rules and outperformed the medical staff at Stanford University. One interesting feature of MYCIN was that it had an NLP interface for both questions and answers. The system also gave explanations for its reasoning (Buchanan and Shortliffe 1984).

10.8.11 IBM Watson Health

IBM Watson Health is an approach by IBM to collect a large amount of information about healthcare in the form of scientific journals, clinical trials, guidelines and textbooks as well as other clinical documents. IBM Watson lets a program index and retrieve, or even interpret, the information and make it available for physicians as answers to their health related questions. IBM Watson Health supports natural language understanding of basic queries that are interpreted and sent to the system. IBM Watson has been used in the areas of cancer kinases and drug repositioning. Cancer kinases, or as the correct term is protein kinases, are enzymes used to treat cancer and drug repositioning is finding a new use for old drugs. The answers are provided as a list of suggestions with a ranking of the closeness or usefulness for the treatment of the patient. The physician will obtain feedback from the system in the form of explanations and the system will also request additional information, as in a dialogue. However, no information has been made available on the performance of the system (Chen et al. 2016; High 2012).

10.9 Summary of Applications of Clinical Text Mining

This chapter has presented a number of applications in clinical text mining as detection and prediction of adverse events such as healthcare associated infections (HAI), and detection of adverse drug events (ADE). Other applications presented were assignment and validation of ICD-10 diagnosis codes for patient records as well as automatic mapping of ICD-10 diagnosis codes to SNOMED CT.

Applications of summarising the patient records were presented, as well as simplification of the patient records for laypeople. An application for generation of patient records text in the neonatal intensive care area was presented.

Search and retrieval techniques for patient records were presented, specifically for cohort studies and comorbidities, along with hypothesis generation using clustering techniques. An information retrieval task, the ShARe/CLEF eHealth Evaluation task for clinical text retrieval was presented, finally classic medical decision (expert) systems such as MYCIN were briefly described, together with IBM Watson Health for assisting the physician in diagnosing the patient.

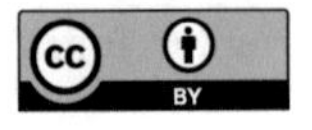

Chapter 11
Networks and Shared Tasks in Clinical Text Mining

Clinical text mining and healthcare text analytics are developed and discussed in several existing researcher networks and practical experiments are carried out in shared tasks. Some of the existing and previous networks are listed below.

- *The Health Natural Language Processing Center (hNLP)*, http://center.healthnlp.org.
- *The UK healthcare text analytics network (Healtex)*, http://healtex.org.
- *The HEalth teXt Analysis network in the Nordic and Baltic countries (HEXAnord)*, http://dsv.su.se/hexanord.
- *The Informatics for Integrating Biology and the Bedside (i2b2)*, https://www.i2b2.org.
- *The Natural Language Processing / Information Extraction (NLP/IE) Program*, https://github.com/nlpie.
- *The Open Health Natural Language Processing Consortium (OHNLP)*, http://www.ohnlp.org/index.php/Main_Page.
- *The Physionet: Multiparameter Intelligent Monitoring in Intensive Care II (MIMIC II) Databases*, https://physionet.org/mimic2/.
  (All links accessed 2018-01-11.)

In these networks both tools and data sets can be found and downloaded for use in clinical text mining.

The shared tasks use clinical text sets that have been made available for the research community. All the data sets have been de-identified and all participants are obliged to sign confidentiality agreements.

The shared tasks are listed below (Huang and Lu 2015).

- *The Computational Medicine Center's (CMC)* 2007 Medical Natural Language Processing Challenge to automatically assign ICD-9 codes to radiology reports.

H. Dalianis, *Clinical Text Mining*, https://doi.org/10.1007/978-3-319-78503-5_11

- *The CoNLL-2018.*[1] Shared task on the detection of sentences containing hedges and in-sentence resolution of hedge cues.
- *i2b2 series of shared tasks from 2010 to 2014.*
  - Extraction of clinical concepts.
  - Identification of clinical relations.
  - Resolution of co-reference.
  - De-identification of clinical discharge summaries.
  - Identification of heart disease risks.
  - Extraction of medication-related information.
  - Reuse of releases, clinical data sets for answering new clinical questions.
  - Prediction of obesity and its co-morbidity.
  - Classification of sentiment at sentence levels.
  - Prediction of smoking status.
  - Evaluation of clinical NLP software usability.
  - Identification of temporal event/expression.
  - Extraction of temporal relation (using the THYME corpora).
- *The Text REtrieval Conference (TREC) Medical,*[2] and Clinical Decision Support (CDS) tracks[3] during 2011–2014.
  - The Medical track treats extraction of cohorts matching inclusion criteria.
  - The CDS track deals with retrieval of relevant documents for clinical decision making and support it is also called the Precision Medicine track.
- The ShARe/CLEF eHealth[4] tasks, which consist of:
  - Normalisation of acronyms/abbreviations.
  - Disease template/attribute filling.
  - Recognition and normalisation of diseases.
  - Retrieval of relevant documents.
  - Interactive search systems for eHealth data.
  - Retrieval of relevant documents for query in different languages.
    (See also Fig. 11.1 for more details on the different ShARe/CLEF eHealth tasks.)
- *The SemEval task in 2014* on the recognition and normalisation of diseases (Pradhan et al. 2014).

---

[1]Overview of the CoNLL-2010 Shared Task, http://rgai.inf.u-szeged.hu/index.php?lang=en&page=conll2010st. Accessed 2018-01-11.

[2]TREC Medical track, http://trec.nist.gov/data/medical.html. Accessed 2018-01-11.

[3]TREC Precision Medicine/Clinical Decision Support Track, http://www.trec-cds.org. Accessed 2018-01-11.

[4]The ShARe/CLEF eHealth tasks https://sites.google.com/site/clefehealth. Accessed 2018-01-11.

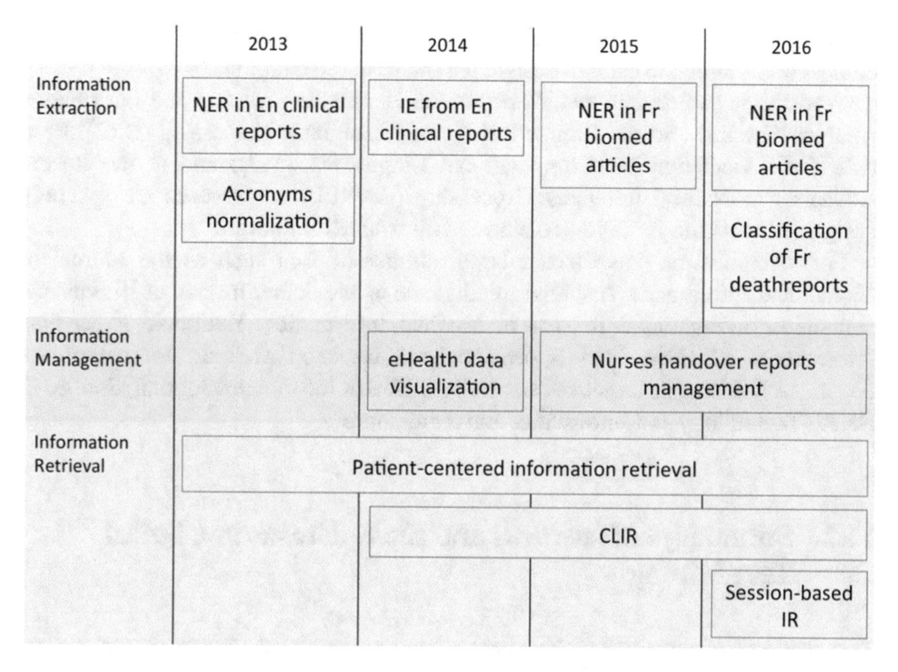

Fig. 11.1 Overview of all ShARe/CLEF eHealth evaluation tasks, from 2013 to 2016,[a] (the figure is courtesy of Hanna Suominen, see Kelly et al. 2016). [a]CLEF eHealth evaluation tasks, https://sites.google.com/site/clefehealth/home/clefehealthtasks.jpg. Accessed 2018-01-11

- *NLP Challenges for Detecting Medication and Adverse Drug Events from Electronic Health Records.*[5]

Many of these shared tasks have been described in this book previously.

In Kelly et al. (2016) all previous ShARe/CLEF eHealth evaluation tasks are mentioned, and specifically for ShARe/CLEF eHealth 2016 all previous shared tasks are repeated. In Fig. 11.1 there is an overview of all ShARe/CLEF eHealth evaluation tasks from 2013 to 2016.

11.1 Conferences, Workshops and Journals

General conferences in natural language processing occasionally contain presentations on clinical text mining. Conferences in health informatics such as the American Medical Informatics Association (AMIA) and Medinfo World Congress

[5]NLP Challenges for Detecting Medication and Adverse Drug Events from Electronic Health Records, http://bio-nlp.org/index.php/announcements/39-nlp-challenges. Accessed 2018-01-11.

on Medical and Health Informatics etc., contain a larger number of articles on clinical text mining, usually in designated tracks at the conferences.

Workshops as International Workshop on Health Text Mining and Information Analysis (Louhi) and the Biomedical Natural Language Processing (BioNLP) at both the Association for Computational Linguistics (ACL) and at the Recent Advances in Natural Language Processing (RANLP) conferences are specially designated workshops in biomedicine and clinical text mining.

For scientific journals there a large number of fora such as the Journal of Biomedical Informatics, Artificial Intelligence in Medicine, Journal of Biomedical Semantics, International Journal of Medical Informatics, Yearbook of Medical Informatics, BMC Medical Informatics and Decision Making, Journal of the American Medical Informatics Association, Health Informatics Journal, Studies in Health Technology and Informatics and many more.

11.2 Summary of Networks and Shared Tasks in Clinical Text Mining

This section has described various networks and shared tasks in the area of clinical text mining and fora for research exchange such as conferences, workshops and scientific journals.

Chapter 12
Conclusions and Outlook

In this book research in clinical text mining from the early days in 1970 up to now (2017) has been compiled. This book provided information on paper based patient record writing as well as the basics in electronic patient records, electronic patient record systems and terminologies. This book described the basic tools for natural language processing of clinical text, including text mining and machine learning techniques and the evaluation of these tools. Lots of examples of applications of clinical text mining have been given.

The book started with the history of the earliest papyrus based patient records in form of instructions for chirurgical treatment of wounds obtained in war in the Ancient Egypt and continued to the father of medicine, Hippocrates, in the Ancient Greece, who took careful notes of the symptoms and treatment of his patients. Hippocrates also urged that these notes should be used by new physicians involved in the treatment of the patients. The Hippocratian way of documenting symptoms and treatment of the diseases was further developed by the Arabs during the Islamic Golden Age, who also introduced hospitals.

In Europe, during the Age of Enlightenment, the taxonomy system of plants and animals was invented by Carl von Linné at Uppsala University. This classification system also inspired to the first classification system of diseases also by Carl von Linné. Nils Rosén von Rosenstein, who was a colleague of Carl von Linné at Uppsala University, introduced and developed the patient record in Sweden.

The book continued with a description of the requirements of electronic patient records systems from the perspective of health personnel, and the development of the electronic patient record systems from the first systems in the 1960s. The transition process from paper based patient records to electronic patient records was also explained.

The book followed with the description of some future support tools for patient record systems, implemented as prototypes assisting the physician and healthcare personnel to obtain a quick overview of the patient record.

H. Dalianis, *Clinical Text Mining*, https://doi.org/10.1007/978-3-319-78503-5_12

The book was continued by pointing at the specific characteristics of the patient record text, such as misspellings, nonstandard abbreviations, jargon and incomplete sentence constructions, the use of Greek and Latin language in the patient records and the different influences of Greek and Latin in Swedish patient record text.

The book followed by presenting the history of the different medical terminology systems, such as ICD diagnosis codes and SNOMED CT, and many other different terminologies and classification systems used in healthcare, for example, ATC drug coding and MeSH for literature indexing.

The challenges in mapping between different terminologies and also how to use ICD-10, SNOMED CT, ATC and MeSH for understanding the meaning of concepts written in free text in patient records have been discussed.

The book described the metrics and methods for evaluating both natural language processing tools and information retrieval tools. For evaluating the tools in a quantitative manner a gold standard is needed, or what in lay language is called "the correct answers". To produce this gold standard manually annotated text was produced; therefore, the manual annotation process for textual data was described as well as the evaluation of the annotation quality.

The annotated data can also be used for the development, training and evaluation of machine learning tools which was described in this book.

The book continued by explaining the basic tools used for natural language processing, and specifically tools adapted for clinical natural language processing. These basic tools included methods for segmentation and tokenisation of string of characters or tokens, the morphological processing of words, such as lemmatisation and stemming, compound splitting, abbreviation detection and expansion. Part-of-speech tagging to reveal the function or word class of each word was explained. Since many words may be misspelled spell checking and spelling correction were also described. To understand the structure of a text syntactical analysis can be carried out, or what is called (syntactical) parsing.

To understand the meaning of a sentence or a text semantical analysis and concept extraction was performed. This was called named entity recognition and negation detection. Negation detection is important since many of the symptoms in clinical text are negated in the reasoning process undertaken by the physician to find the disorder of the patient. Part of the semantic analysis consisted of processing steps to find relations between a drug and its effect or side effect. This was called relation extraction and more research is still needed on obtaining valuable results.

Clinical text also contains many temporal expressions that need to be resolved to understand when something occurred in a time line in the discourse. Therefore, tools have been developed to process temporality. These temporal processing tools were described and the different frameworks that were developed to deal with temporality in clinical text were explained.

Computational methods such as rule-based methods and machine learning methods were described, their differences and their pros and cons. Different ready-to-use tools were demonstrated. Since manual annotation of clinical text is costly (as well as all annotation work in general), active learning has been developed. Active learning assists in choosing the most optimal and useful data for annotation such that is reduced annotation time.

To obtain electronic patient records for research ethical permission was needed. The process of applying ethical permission was explained. Ethics and privacy for the access and use of electronic patient records were discussed as well as the safe storage of the electronic patient records.

De-identification and pseudonymisation of sensitive data in electronic patient records text was described. Sensitive data is mostly data that can identify individuals, usually this data was either removed, by removing the whole data table that contained the sensitive data, or by anonymising the data in the data table. However, the sensitive data is often present in the clinical free text in form of names, addresses and telephone numbers, which need to be automatically identified and then removed, or pseudonymised which means to change the names to fake names or surrogates, the addresses to pseudo addresses etc.

The final main chapter presented a series of useful applications using the patient record data as input to these applications. Applications ranging from the presentation of the patient records in the form of an automatic summary to presentation of the basic concepts in patient record in the form of automatically extracted key words to support for the production of patient records text in the form of spelling correction systems, to big data analytics in the form of adverse event and healthcare associated infection detection and prediction. Natural language generation to produce useful text from various data that can be used by clinicians was also presented, including generation of natural language descriptions of SNOMED CT concepts. Other useful applications are comorbidity networks to find which disease co-occur or causes other diseases and various methods for hypothesis generation from clinical texts.

Various retrieval methods to extracts cohorts of patients with certain characteristics which is also an important domain were presented in the book. Using the clinical text as input for detecting adverse drug events, healthcare associated infections, pressure sores, patient falls, device failures, nutrition problems and surgical complication are also important and was presented in this textbook. Various clinical decision systems were presented as well as tools for automatic ICD to SNOMED CT mapping. One speech application was also presented to make early detection of dementia on patients.

The book ended with a presentation of the number of research networks and performed shared tasks in the clinical text mining.

At the beginning of the book a number of research questions were posed that are answered below:

- One main research question is: *Using artificial intelligence to analyse patient records: is it possible and will it improve healthcare?* The answer will be yes, if Artificial Intelligence is considered as a smart algorithm that will support humans and not as an independent will with a *soul* or a *deterministic will*.
- Another research question, which is rather long, is: *Can one process clinical text written in Swedish with natural language processing tools developed for standard Swedish such as newspaper and web texts, to extract named entities such as*

symptoms, diagnosis, drugs and body parts from clinical text? This question can partly be answered as yes, but of course since patient record texts are very domain specific this can not be carried out with the standard NLP tools, instead tools need to be adapted to the clinical domain.

Then followed a number of research sub questions as:

- Can one decide the factuality of a diagnosis found in a clinical text? What does *Pneumonia?* or *Angina pectoris cannot be excluded* or just *No signs of pneumonia?* really mean? The answer to this question is yes, to a certain level this can be carried out.
- *Can one determine of the temporal order of clinical events? Have the symptoms occurred a week ago or two years ago?* The answer is not completely yes, since it is difficult to extract temporal relations from free text and to align relative and absolute time points.
- *Can new adverse drug effects be found by extracting relations between drug intake and adverse drug effect?* The answer is no, the surveillance systems using clinical texts have not found new adverse drug effects yet, but this is a question of time and it will soon happen.
- *How much clinical text must be annotated manually to obtain correct and useful results?* The answer is probably at least 5000 annotated entities for NER, the proposed number of annotations gives usually rather good results after training. Regarding the task of relation extraction this is difficult to say, since the results are rather poor.
- *How can patient privacy be maintained while carrying out research in clinical text mining?* This is a difficult question to answer since the more data we leave behind traces on the different public digital places and business systems the easier it will be to track citizens, and our information can then be used to break privacy.

This book will probably become the standard text book for another 10 years until is updated by another textbook in the clinical text mining area.

This book has collected a vast amount of knowledge in the area clinical text mining combined with healthcare analytics and medicine. The knowledge was presented in a pedagogical and didactic way, explaining healthcare concepts. Healthcare concepts are described in the context of natural language processing and text mining methods. This book has leveraged future research and development of useful applications for healthcare. This was carried out by enabling the unlocking of previous knowledge and experience of thousands of clinicians, such as physicians and nurses, which was documented in thousands of electronic patient record repositories throughout the world. This unlocked knowledge will improve healthcare for humanity.

12.1 Outcomes

The book will become the standard scientific book for clinical text mining. The research results will be linked to courses at DSV, the Stockholm University, along with Master's in Health informatics that is jointly administered by Karolinska Institute and Stockholm University. Karolinska University Hospital, Stockholm County Council (SLL), other county councils in Sweden and companies such as Capish Knowledge and IMS Health Sweden, now IQVIA, are other stakeholders of this book.

References

Afzal, Z., Pons, E., Kang, N., Sturkenboom, M. C. J. M., Schuemie, M. J., & Kors, J. A. (2014). ContextD: An algorithm to identify contextual properties of medical terms in a Dutch clinical corpus. *BMC Bioinformatics, 15*(1), 373.

Agrawal, R., & Srikant, R. (1994). Fast algorithms for mining association rules. In *Proceedings 20th International Conference on Very Large Data Bases, VLDB* (Vol. 1215, pp. 487–499).

Åhlfeldt, H., Borin, L., Grabar, N., Hallett, C., Hardcastle, D., Kokkinakis, D., et al. (2006). *Literature Review on Patient-Friendly Documentation Systems.* Technical report, Network of Excellence Semantic Mining, Work Package 27 Deliverable 1.

Ahltorp, M., Skeppstedt, M., Kitajima, S., Rzepka, R., & Araki, K. (2014). Medical vocabulary mining using distributional semantics on Japanese patient blogs. In *6th International Symposium on Semantic Mining in Biomedicine (SMBM), Aveiro, Portugal, October 6–7, 2014* (pp. 57–62).

Al-Awqati, Q. (2006). How to write a case report: Lessons from 1600 BC. *Kidney International, 69*(12), 2113–2114.

Alfalahi, A., Brissman, S., & Dalianis, H. (2012). Pseudonymisation of personal names and other PHIs in an annotated clinical Swedish corpus. In *Third Workshop on Building and Evaluating Resources for Biomedical Text Mining (BioTxtM 2012) Held in Conjunction with LREC 2012, May 26, Istanbul* (pp. 49–54).

Alfalahi, A., Skeppstedt, M., Ahlbom, R., Baskalayci, R., Henriksson, A., Asker, L., et al. (2015). Expanding a dictionary of marker words for uncertainty and negation using distributional semantics. In *Proceedings of the Sixth International Workshop on Health Text Mining and Information Analysis, Louhi, Held in Conjunction with EMNLP 2015, Lisbon, Portugal* (pp. 90–96). Association for Computational Linguistics.

Allen, J. F. (1984). Towards a general theory of action and time. *Artificial Intelligence, 23*(2), 123–154.

Allvin, H., Carlsson, E., Dalianis, H., Danielsson-Ojala, R., Daudaravicius, V., Hassel, M., et al. (2011). Characteristics of Finnish and Swedish intensive care nursing narratives: A comparative analysis to support the development of clinical language technologies. *Journal of Biomedical Semantics, 2*(Suppl 3), 1–11.

Almgren, S., & Pavlov, S. (2016). *Semi-supervised Named Entity Recognition of Medical Entities in Swedish.* Master's thesis, Department of Computer Science and Engineering, Chalmers University of Technology.

Almgren, S., Pavlov, S., & Mogren, O. (2016). Named entity recognition in Swedish health records with character-based deep bidirectional LSTMs. In *Proceedings of the Fifth Workshop on Building and Evaluating Resources for Biomedical Text Mining (BioTxtM 2016), Held in Conjunction with Coling 2016* (pp. 30–29).

H. Dalianis, *Clinical Text Mining*, https://doi.org/10.1007/978-3-319-78503-5

Alpaydin, E. (2014). *Introduction to Machine Learning*. Cambridge, MA: The MIT Press.

Andersen, A., Yigzaw, K. Y., & Karlsen, R. (2014). Privacy preserving health data processing. In *2014 IEEE 16th International Conference on e-Health Networking, Applications and Services (Healthcom)* (pp. 225–230). New York: IEEE.

Andersson, P., & Sjöberg, A. (2016). *Generating and Evaluating an Automatic Mapping Between SNOMED-CT and the Swedish Extension Codes of ICD-10 Based on Lexical Similarities*. Master's thesis, Department of Computer and Systems Sciences, Stockholm University.

Antfolk, A., & Branting, R. (2016). *Pseudonymisering av platser i patient-journaltexter (In Swedish)*. Bachelor's thesis, Department of Computer and Systems Sciences, Stockholm University.

Aramaki, E., Miura, Y., Tonoike, M., Ohkuma, T., Mashuichi, H., & Ohe, K. (2009). Text2table: Medical text summarization system based on named entity recognition and modality identification. In *Proceedings of the Workshop on Current Trends in Biomedical Natural Language Processing* (pp. 185–192). Association for Computational Linguistics.

Aramaki, E., Miura, Y., Tonoike, M., Ohkuma, T., Masuichi, H., Waki, K., et al. (2010). Extraction of adverse drug effects from clinical records. *Studies in Health Technology and Informatics, 160*(Pt 1), 739–743.

Aramaki, E., Morita, M., Kano, Y., & Ohkuma, T. (2014). Overview of the NTCIR-11 MedNLP-2 Task. In *NTCIR*.

Artstein, R., & Poesio, M. (2008). Inter-coder agreement for computational linguistics. *Computational Linguistics, 34*(4), 555–596.

Asamura, H., Wittekind, C., & Sobin, L. H. (2014). *TNM Atlas: Illustrated Guide to the TNM Classification of Malignant Tumours*. New York: Wiley.

Attardi, G., Cozza, V., & Sartiano, D. (2015). Annotation and extraction of relations from Italian medical records. In *Proceedings of the 6th Italian Information Retrieval Workshop, Cagliari, Italy*.

Bagga, A., & Baldwin, B. (1998). Algorithms for scoring coreference chains. In *The First International Conference on Language Resources and Evaluation Workshop on Linguistics Coreference, Granada, Spain* (Vol. 1, pp. 563–566).

Bailey, C., Peddie, D., Wickham, M. E., Badke, K., Small, S. S., Doyle-Waters, M. M., et al. (2016). Adverse drug event reporting systems: A systematic review. *British Journal of Clinical Pharmacology, 82*(1), 17–29.

Bank, M., & Schierle, M. (2012). A survey of text mining architectures and the UIMA Standard. In *Proceedings of the Eighth International Conference on Language Resources and Evaluation, LREC 2012* (pp. 3479–3486).

Barak-Corren, Y., Castro, V. M., Javitt, S., Hoffnagle, A. G., Dai, Y., Perlis, R. H., et al. (2016). Predicting suicidal behavior from longitudinal electronic health records. *American Journal of Psychiatry, 174*(2), 154–162.

Beijer, H. J. M., & de Blaey, C. J. (2002). Hospitalisations caused by adverse drug reactions (ADR): A meta-analysis of observational studies. *Pharmacy World and Science, 24*(2), 46–54.

Bejan, C. A., & Denny, J. C. (2014). Learning to identify treatment relations in clinical text. In *AMIA Annual Symposium Proceedings* (Vol. 2014, p. 282). American Medical Informatics Association.

Björkegren, A. (2011). *Pseudonymisering av digitala patientjournaler (In Swedish)*. Bachelor's thesis, Department of Computer and Systems Sciences, Stockholm University.

Blacky, A., Mandl, H., Adlassnig, K.-P., & Koller, W. (2011). Fully automated surveillance of healthcare-associated infections with MONI-ICU - A Breakthrough in clinical infection surveillance. *Applied Clinical Informatics, 2*(3), 365–372.

Blei, D. M. (2012). Probabilistic topic models. *Communications of the ACM, 55*(4), 77–84.

Boström, H., & Dalianis, H. (2012). De-identifying health records by means of active learning. In *Proceedings of the 29th International Conference on Machine Learning ICML 2012* (pp. 1–3).

Boytcheva, S. (2011). Automatic matching of ICD-10 codes to diagnoses in discharge letters. In *Proceedings of the Workshop on Biomedical Natural Language Processing* (pp. 11–18).

Boytcheva, S., Angelova, G., Angelov, Z., & Tcharaktchiev, D. (2015). Text mining and big data analytics for retrospective analysis of clinical texts from outpatient care. *Cybernetics and Information Technologies, 15*(4), 58–77.

Boytcheva, S., Nikolova, I., & Angelova, G. (2017a). Mining association rules from clinical narratives. In *Proceedings of Recent Advances in Natural Language Processing, RANLP 2017, Varna, Bulgaria* (pp. 130–138).

Boytcheva, S., Nikolova, I., Angelova, G., & Angelov, Z. (2017b). Identification of risk factors in clinical texts through association rules. In *Proceedings of RANLP Workshop on Biomedical Natural Language Processing* (pp. 64–72).

Buchanan, B. G., & Shortliffe, E. H. (1984). *Rule-Based Expert Systems* (Vol. 3). Reading, MA: Addison-Wesley.

Buckley, J. M., Coopey, S. B., Sharko, J., Polubriaginof, F., Drohan, B., Belli, A. K., et al. (2012). The feasibility of using natural language processing to extract clinical information from breast pathology reports. *Journal of Pathology Informatics, 3*(1), 23.

Cameron, S., & Turtle-Song, I. (2002). Learning to write case notes using the SOAP format. *Journal of Counseling and Development, 80*(3), 286.

Carlberger, J., Dalianis, H., Hassel, M., & Knutsson, O. (2001). Improving precision in information retrieval for Swedish using stemming. In *Proceedings of NODALIDA '01 - 13th Nordic Conference on Computational Linguistics*.

Carrell, D., Malin, B., Aberdeen, J., Bayer, S., Clark, C., Wellner, B., et al. (2013). Hiding in plain sight: Use of realistic surrogates to reduce exposure of protected health information in clinical text. *Journal of the American Medical Informatics Association, 20*(2), 342–348.

Casillas, A., Pérez, A., Oronoz, M., Gojenola, K., & Santiso, S. (2016). Learning to extract adverse drug reaction events from electronic health records in Spanish. *Expert Systems with Applications, 61*, 235–245.

Cederblom, S. (2005). *Medicinska förkortningar och akronymer*. Studentlitteratur, Lund.

Chapman, W. W., Bridewell, W., Hanbury, P., Cooper, G. F., & Buchanan, B. G. (2001). A simple algorithm for identifying negated findings and diseases in discharge summaries. *Journal of Biomedical Informatics, 34*(5), 301–310.

Chapman, W. W., Hilert, D., Velupillai, S., Kvist, M., Skeppstedt, M., Chapman, B. E., et al. (2013). Extending the NegEx lexicon for multiple languages. *Studies in Health Technology and Informatics, 192*, 677.

Chazard, E., Ficheur, G., Bernonville, S., Luyckx, M., & Beuscart, R. (2011). Data mining to generate adverse drug events detection rules. *IEEE Transactions on Information Technology in Biomedicine, 15*(6), 823–830.

Chen, R., & Klein, G. (2007). The openEHR Java reference implementation project. *Studies in Health Technology and Informatics, 129*(1), 58.

Chen, R., Klein, G. O., Sundvall, E., Karlsson, D., & Åhlfeldt, H. (2009). Archetype-based conversion of EHR content models: Pilot experience with a regional EHR system. *BMC Medical Informatics and Decision Making, 9*(1), 33.

Chen, Y., Argentinis, J. D. E., & Weber, G. (2016). IBM Watson: How cognitive computing can be applied to big data challenges in life sciences research. *Clinical Therapeutics, 38*(4), 688–701.

Cheng, T. O. (2001). Hippocrates and cardiology. *American Heart Journal, 141*(2), 173–183.

Chinchor, N., & Robinson, P. (1997). MUC-7 named entity task definition. In *Proceedings of the 7th Conference on Message Understanding* (p. 29).

Clark, A., Fox, C., & Lappin, S. (2013). *The Handbook of Computational Linguistics and Natural Language Processing*. New York: Wiley.

Cleverdon, C. (1967). The Cranfield tests on index language devices. In *Aslib Proceedings* (pp. 173–194). MCB UP Ltd.

Coden, A., Savova, G., Sominsky, I., Tanenblatt, M., Masanz, J., Schuler, K., et al. (2009). Automatically extracting cancer disease characteristics from pathology reports into a disease knowledge representation model. *Journal of Biomedical Informatics, 42*(5), 937–949.

Cohen, K. B., & Demner-Fushman, D. (2014). *Biomedical Natural Language Processing* (Vol. 11). Amsterdam: John Benjamins Publishing Company.

Costumero, R., Lopez, F., Gonzalo-Martín, C., Millan, M., & Menasalvas, E. (2014). An approach to detect negation on medical documents in Spanish. In *International Conference on Brain Informatics and Health* (pp. 366–375). Berlin: Springer.

Cotik, V., Filippo, D., Uszkoreit, H., & Xu, F. (2017). Annotation of entities and relations in Spanish radiology reports. In *Proceedings of Recent Advances in Natural Language Processing, RANLP 2017, Varna, Bulgaria* (pp. 177–184).

Cotik, V., Roller, R., Xu, F., Uszkoreit, H., Budde, K., & Schmidt, D. (2016). Negation detection in clinical reports written in German. *In the Proceedings of the Fifth Workshop on Building and Evaluating Resources for Biomedical Text Mining (BioTxtM 2016), Held in Conjunction with Coling 2016* (pp. 115–124).

Currie, A.-M., Fricke, T., Gawne, A., Johnston, R., Liu, J., & Stein, B. (2006). Automated extraction of free-text from pathology reports. In *AMIA Annual Symposium Proceedings*.

Dahl, A., Özkan, A., & Dalianis, H. (2016). Pathology text mining-on Norwegian prostate cancer reports. In *2016 IEEE 32nd International Conference on Data Engineering Workshops (ICDEW)* (pp. 84–87). New York: IEEE.

Dalianis, H. (2014). Clinical text retrieval - An overview of basic building blocks and applications. In *Professional Search in the Modern World* (pp. 147–165). Berlin: Springer.

Dalianis, H., & Boström, H. (2012). Releasing a Swedish clinical corpus after removing all words–de-identification experiments with conditional random fields and random forests. In *Proceedings of the Third Workshop on Building and Evaluating Resources for Biomedical Text Mining (BioTxtM 2012) Held in Conjunction with LREC* (pp. 45–48).

Dalianis, H., Hassel, M., & Velupillai, S. (2009). The Stockholm EPR Corpus-characteristics and some initial findings. In *Proceedings of ISHIMR 2009, Evaluation and Implementation of e-Health and Health Information Initiatives: International Perspectives. 14th International Symposium for Health Information Management Research* (pp. 243–249).

Dalianis, H., Henriksson, A., Kvist, M., Velupillai, S., & Weegar, R. (2015). HEALTH BANK–A workbench for data science applications in healthcare. In J. Krogstie, G. Juel-Skielse, & V. Kabilan (Eds.), *Proceedings of the CAiSE-2015 Industry Track Co-located with 27th Conference on Advanced Information Systems Engineering (CAiSE 2015), Stockholm, Sweden, June 11, 2015, CEUR* (Vol. 1381, pp. 1–18). https://doi.org/urn:nbn:de:0074-1381-0E.

Dalianis, H., & Skeppstedt, M. (2010). Creating and evaluating a consensus for negated and speculative words in a Swedish clinical corpus. In *Proceedings of the Workshop on Negation and Speculation in Natural Language Processing* (pp. 5–13). Association for Computational Linguistics.

Dalianis, H., & Velupillai, S. (2010a). How certain are clinical assessments? Annotating Swedish clinical text for (un) certainties, speculations and negations. In *Proceedings of the Seventh International Conference on Language Resources and Evaluation, LREC 2010*.

Dalianis, H., & Velupillai, S. (2010b). De-identifying Swedish clinical text-refinement of a gold standard and experiments with conditional random fields. *Journal of Biomedical Semantics, 1*, 6.

Damerau, F. J. (1964). A technique for computer detection and correction of spelling errors. *Communications of the ACM, 7*(3), 171–176.

de Bruijn, B., Cherry, C., Kiritchenko, S., Martin, J., & Zhu, X. (2011). Machine-learned solutions for three stages of clinical information extraction: The state of the art at i2b2 2010. *Journal of the American Medical Informatics Association, 18*(5), 557–562.

Decker, A. (2003). *Towards Automatic Grammatical Simplification of Swedish Text*. Master's thesis, Computational Linguistics, Department of Linguistics, Stockholm University.

Deleger, L., Lingren, T., Ni, Y., Kaiser, M., Stoutenborough, L., Marsolo, K., et al. (2014). Preparing an annotated gold standard corpus to share with extramural investigators for de-identification research. *Journal of Biomedical Informatics, 50*, 173–183.

Derczynski, L. R. A. (2017). *Automatically Ordering Events and Times in Text*. Berlin: Springer.

Doan, S., Bastarache, L., Klimkowski, S., Denny, J. C., & Xu, H. (2010). Integrating existing natural language processing tools for medication extraction from discharge summaries. *Journal of the American Medical Informatics Association, 17*(5), 528–531.

Dorr, D. A., Phillips, W. F., Phansalkar, S., Sims, S. A., & Hurdle, J. F. (2006). Assessing the difficulty and time cost of de-identification in clinical narratives. *Methods of Information in Medicine, 45*(3), 246–252.

Douglass, M., Clifford, G. D., Reisner, A., Moody, G. B., & Mark, R. G. (2004). Computer-assisted de-identification of free text in the MIMIC II database. In *Computers in Cardiology, 2004* (pp. 341–344). New York: IEEE.

Doupi, P., Svaar, H., Bjørn, B., Deilkås, E., Nylén, U., & Rutberg, H. (2015). Use of the global trigger tool in patient safety improvement efforts: Nordic experiences. *Cognition, Technology & Work, 17*(1), 45–54.

Downs, J., Velupillai, S., Gkotsis, G., Holden, R., Kikoler, M., Dean, H., et al. (2017). Detection of suicidality in adolescents with autism spectrum disorders: Developing a natural language processing approach for use in electronic health records. In *AMIA Annual Symposium Proceedings*.

Ducel, G., Fabry, J., & Nicolle, L. (Eds.). (2002). *Prevention of Hospital Acquired Infections: A Practical Guide.*, 2nd edn. World Health Organization. http://www.who.int/csr/resources/publications/drugresist/WHO_CDS_CSR_EPH_2002_12/en/. Accessed 11 Jan 2018.

Dziadek, J. (2015). *Improving SNOMED Mapping of Clinical Texts Using Context-Sensitive Spelling Correction*. Master's thesis, Department of Computer and Systems Sciences, Stockholm University.

Dziadek, J., Henriksson, A., & Duneld, M. (2017). Improving terminology mapping in clinical text with context-sensitive spelling correction. *Informatics for Health: Connected Citizen-Led Wellness and Population Health, 235*, 241.

Edwards, I. R., & Aronson, J. K. (2000). Adverse drug reactions: Definitions, diagnosis, and management. *The Lancet, 356*(9237), 1255–1259.

Ehrentraut, C., Ekholm, M., Tanushi, H., Tiedemann, J., & Dalianis, H. (2016). Detecting hospital-acquired infections: A document classification approach using support vector machines and gradient tree boosting. *Health Informatics Journal, 24*(1), 24–42.

Ehrentraut, C., Kvist, M., Sparrelid, E., & Dalianis, H. (2014). Detecting healthcare-associated infections in electronic health records: Evaluation of machine learning and preprocessing techniques. In *Sixth International Symposium on Semantic Mining in Biomedicine (SMBM 2014)*. University of Aveiro.

Ehrentraut, C., Tanushi, H., Tiedemann, J., & Dalianis, H. (2012). Detection of hospital acquired infections in sparse and noisy Swedish patient records. In *Proceedings of the Sixth Workshop on Analytics for Noisy Unstructured Text Data (AND 2012) Held in Conjunction with Coling 2012, Bombay*. ACM Digital Library.

El Emam, K., Rodgers, S., & Malin, B. (2015). Anonymising and sharing individual patient data. *BMJ, 350*, h1139.

Elhadad, N., McKeown, K., Kaufman, D. R., & Jordan, D. A. (2005). Facilitating physicians' access to information via tailored text summarization. In *AMIA Annual Symposium Proceedings*. Citeseer.

Eriksson, R., Jensen, P. B., Frankild, S., Jensen, L. J., & Brunak, S. (2013). Dictionary construction and identification of possible adverse drug events in Danish clinical narrative text. *Journal of the American Medical Informatics Association, 20*(5), 947–953.

Falkenjack, J., Fahlborg, D., Rennes, E., Johansson, V., & Jönsson, A. (2017). Services for text simplification and analysis. In *Proceedings of NODALIDA '17 - 21th Nordic Conference on Computational Linguistics*.

Farkas, R., & Szarvas, G. (2008). Automatic construction of rule-based ICD-9-CM coding systems. *BMC Bioinformatics, 9*(3), S10.

Forster, A. J., Jennings, A., Chow, C., Leeder, C., & van Walraven, C. (2012). A systematic review to evaluate the accuracy of electronic adverse drug event detection. *Journal of the American Medical Informatics Association, 19*(1), 31–38.

Fraser, K. C., Meltzer, J. A., & Rudzicz, F. (2015). Linguistic features identify Alzheimer's disease in narrative speech. *Journal of Alzheimer's Disease, 49*(2), 407–422.

Freeman, R., Moore, L. S. P., Álvarez, L. G., Charlett, A., & Holmes, A. (2013). Advances in electronic surveillance for healthcare-associated infections in the 21st century: A systematic review. *Journal of Hospital Infection, 84*(2), 106–119.

Friedman, C. (2005). Semantic text parsing for patient records. In *Medical Informatics* (pp. 423–448). Berlin: Springer.

Friedman, C., & Hripcsak, G. (1999). Natural language processing and its future in medicine. *Academic Medicine, 74*(8), 890–895.

Friedman, C., Johnson, S. B., Forman, B., & Starren, J. (1995). Architectural requirements for a multipurpose natural language processor in the clinical environment. In *Proceedings of the Annual Symposium on Computer Application in Medical Care* (p. 347). American Medical Informatics Association.

Friedrich, S., & Dalianis, H. (2015). Adverse drug event classification of health records using dictionary-based pre-processing and machine learning. In *Proceedings of the Sixth International Workshop on Health Text Mining and Information Analysis, Louhi, Held in Conjunction with EMNLP 2015, Lisbon, Portugal* (pp. 121–130).

Garrett, L. E., Hammond, W. E., & Stead, W. W. (1986). The effects of computerized medical records on provider efficiency and quality of care. *Methods of Information in Medicine, 25*(3), 151–157.

Gerdes, L. U., & Hardahl, C. (2012). Text mining electronic health records to identify hospital adverse events. *Studies in Health Technology and Informatics, 192*, 1145–1145.

Gillum, R. F. (2013). From papyrus to the electronic tablet: A brief history of the clinical medical record with lessons for the digital age. *The American Journal of Medicine, 126*(10), 853–857.

Gkotsis, G., Velupillai, S., Oellrich, A., Dean, H., Liakata, M., & Dutta, R. (2016). Don't let notes be misunderstood: A negation detection method for assessing risk of suicide in mental health records. In *Proceedings of the 3rd Workshop on Computational Linguistics and Clinical Psychology: From Linguistic Signal to Clinical Reality* (pp. 95–105). Association for Computational Linguistics.

Gkoulalas-Divanis, A., Loukides, G., & Sun, J. (2014). Publishing data from electronic health records while preserving privacy: A survey of algorithms. *Journal of Biomedical Informatics, 50*, 4–19.

Grigonyte, G., Kvist, M., Velupillai, S., & Wirén, M. Improving readability of Swedish electronic health records through lexical simplification: First results. In *Proceedings of the 3rd Workshop on Predicting and Improving Text Readability for Target Reader Populations – PITR*, Gothenburg, Sweden, April 2014 (pp. 74–83). Association for Computational Linguistics. http://www.aclweb.org/anthology/W14-1209. Accessed 11 Jan 2018.

Grigonytė, G., Kvist, M., Wirén, M., Velupillai, S., & Henriksson, A. (2016). Swedification patterns of Latin and Greek affixes in clinical text. *Nordic Journal of Linguistics, 39*(01), 5–37.

Groopman, J. E. (2007). *How Doctors Think*. New York: Houghton Mifflin Company.

Grouin, C., Deléger, L., Rosier, A., Temal, L., Dameron, O., Van Hille, P., et al. (2011). Automatic computation of CHA2DS2-VASc score: Information extraction from clinical texts for thromboembolism risk assessment. In *AMIA Annual Symposium Proceedings* (pp. 501–510). American Medical Informatics Association.

Grouin, C., & Névéol, A. (2014). De-identification of clinical notes in French: Towards a protocol for reference corpus development. *Journal of Biomedical Informatics, 50*, 151–161.

Gurulingappa, H., Rajput, A. M., Roberts, A., Fluck, J., Hofmann-Apitius, M., & Toldo, L. (2012). Development of a benchmark corpus to support the automatic extraction of drug-related adverse effects from medical case reports. *Journal of Biomedical Informatics, 45*(5), 885–892.

Haerian, K., Salmasian, H., & Friedman, C. (2012). Methods for identifying suicide or suicidal ideation in EHRs. In *AMIA Annual Symposium Proceedings* (Vol. 2012, p. 1244). American Medical Informatics Association.

Halpin, H., Shortell, S. M., Milstein, A., & Vanneman, M. (2011). Hospital adoption of automated surveillance technology and the implementation of infection prevention and control programs. *American Journal of Infection Control, 39*(4), 270–276.

Hamon, T., & Grabar, N. (2014). Tuning HeidelTime for identifying time expressions in clinical texts in English and French. In *Proceedings of the 5th International Workshop on Health Text Mining and Information Analysis (Louhi)@ EACL* (pp. 101–105). Citeseer.
Hanauer, D., Aberdeen, J., Bayer, S., Wellner, B., Clark, C., Zheng, K., & Hirschman, L. (2013). Bootstrapping a de-identification system for narrative patient records: Cost-performance tradeoffs. *International Journal of Medical Informatics, 82*(9), 821–831.
Harkema, H., Dowling, J. N., Thornblade, T., & Chapman, W. W. (2009). ConText: An algorithm for determining negation, experiencer, and temporal status from clinical reports. *Journal of Biomedical Informatics, 42*(5), 839–851.
Harpaz, R., DuMouchel, W., Shah, N. H., Madigan, D., Ryan, P., & Friedman, C. (2012). Novel data-mining methodologies for adverse drug event discovery and analysis. *Clinical Pharmacology & Therapeutics, 91*(6), 1010–1021.
Hassel, M. (2007). *Resource Lean and Portable Automatic Text Summarization*. PhD thesis, School of Computer Science and Communication, Royal Institute of Technology, Stockholm, Sweden, June 2007. http://nlp.lacasahassel.net/publications/hasselthesis07phd.pdf. Accessed 11 Jan 2018.
Hassel, M., Henriksson, A., & Velupillai, S. (2011). Something old, something new: Applying a pre-trained parsing model to clinical Swedish. In *Northern European Association for Language Technology (NEALT)*.
Hassel, M., & Sjöbergh, J. (2006). Towards holistic summarization: Selecting summaries, not sentences. In *Proceedings of LREC 2006*, Genoa, Italy. http://nlp.lacasahassel.net/publications/holsum06.pdf. Accessed 11 Jan 2018.
Hazlehurst, B., Naleway, A., & Mullooly, J. (2009). Detecting possible vaccine adverse events in clinical notes of the electronic medical record. *Vaccine, 27*(14), 2077–2083.
He, T. Y. (2007). *Coreference Resolution on Entities and Events for Hospital Discharge Summaries*. Master's thesis, Electrical Engineering and Computer Science, Massachusetts Institute of Technology.
Health Insurance Portability and Accountability Act (HIPAA). (2003). U.S. Department of Health and Human Services. http://www.cdc.gov/mmwr/preview/mmwrhtml/m2e411a1.htm. Accessed 11 Jan 2018.
Henriksson, A. (2015). *Ensembles of Semantic Spaces, on Combining Models of Distributional Semantics with Applications in Healthcare*. PhD thesis, Department of Computer and Systems Sciences, Stockholm University.
Henriksson, A., & Hassel, M. (2013). Optimizing the dimensionality of clinical term spaces for improved diagnosis coding support. In *Proceedings of Louhi Workshop on Health Document Text Mining and Information Analysis*.
Henriksson, A., Hassel, M., & Kvist, M. (2011). Diagnosis code assignment support using random indexing of patient records – A qualitative feasibility study. In *Proceedings of Artificial Intelligence in Medicine* (pp. 348–352). Berlin: Springer.
Henriksson, A., Kvist, M., & Dalianis, H. (2017a). Prevalence estimation of protected health information in Swedish clinical text. Studies in Health Technology and Informatics, Vol 235, pp. 216–220.
Henriksson, A., Kvist, M., & Dalianis, H. (2017b). Detecting protected health information in heterogeneous clinical notes. Studies in Health Technology and Informatics, Vol 245, pp. 394–397.
Henriksson, A., Kvist, M., Dalianis, H., & Duneld, M. (2015). Identifying adverse drug event information in clinical notes with distributional semantic representations of context. *Journal of Biomedical Informatics, 57*, 333–349.
Henriksson, A., Moen, H., Skeppstedt, M., Daudaravicius, V., & Duneld, M. (2014). Synonym extraction and abbreviation expansion with ensembles of semantic spaces. *Journal of Biomedical Semantics, 5*, 6.
High, R. (2012). *The Era of Cognitive Systems: An Inside Look at IBM Watson and How it Works*. IBM Corporation, Redbooks.

Hripcsak, G., & Rothschild, A. S. (2005). Agreement, the F-measure, and reliability in information retrievas. *Journal of the American Medical Informatics Association, 12*(3), 296–298.

Huang, C.-C., & Lu, Z. (2015). Community challenges in biomedical text mining over 10 years: Success, failure and the future. *Briefings in Bioinformatics, 17*(1), 132–144.

Huang, Y., & Lowe, H. J. (2007). A novel hybrid approach to automated negation detection in clinical radiology reports. *Journal of the American Medical Informatics Association, 14*(3), 304.

Humphreys, B. L., Lindberg, D. A. B., Schoolman, H. M., & Barnett, G. O. (1998). The unified medical language system. *Journal of the American Medical Informatics Association, 5*(1), 1–11.

Humphreys, H., & Smyth, E. T. M. (2006). Prevalence surveys of healthcare-associated infections: What do they tell us, if anything? *Clinical Microbiology and Infection, 12*(1), 2–4.

IHTSDO. (2016). SNOMED-CT, Systematized nomenclature of medicine-clinical terms. http://www.ihtsdo.org/snomed-ct/. Accessed 11 Jan 2018.

Isenius, N. (2012). *Abbreviation Detection in Swedish Medical Records. The Development of SCAN, A Swedish Clinical Abbreviation Normalizer*. Master's thesis, Department of Computer and Systems Sciences, Stockholm University.

Isenius, N., Velupillai, S., & Kvist, M. (2012). Initial results in the development of SCAN. A Swedish clinical abbreviation normalizer. In *CLEFeHealth 2012 Workshop on Cross-Language Evaluation of Methods, Applications, and Resources for eHealth Document Analysis, Rome*.

Jacobson, O., & Dalianis, H. (2016). Applying deep learning on electronic health records in Swedish to predict healthcare-associated infections. In *ACL Proceedings of the 15th Workshop on Biomedical Natural Language Processing, BioNLP 2016* (pp. 191–195).

Japkowicz, N., & Shah, M. (2011). *Evaluating Learning Algorithms: A Classification Perspective*. Cambridge: Cambridge University Press.

Jensen, K., Soguero-Ruiz, C., Mikalsen, K. O., Lindsetmo, R.-O., Kouskoumvekaki, I., Girolami, M., et al. (2017). Analysis of free text in electronic health records for identification of cancer patient trajectories. *Scientific Reports, 7*, 46226.

Jensen, P. B., Jensen, L. J., & Brunak, S. (2012). Mining electronic health records: Towards better research applications and clinical care. *Nature Reviews Genetics, 13*(6), 395–405.

Jiang, M., Chen, Y., Liu, M., Rosenbloom, S. T., Mani, S., Denny, J. C., et al. (2011). A study of machine-learning-based approaches to extract clinical entities and their assertions from discharge summaries. *Journal of the American Medical Informatics Association, 18*(5), 601–606.

Johnson, S. B., Bakken, S., Dine, D., Hyun, S., Mendonça, E., Morrison, F., et al. (2008). An electronic health record based on structured narrative. *Journal of the American Medical Informatics Association, 15*(1), 54–64.

Jung, H., Allen, J., Blaylock, N., De Beaumont, W., Galescu, L., & Swift, M. (2011). Building timelines from narrative clinical records: Initial results based-on deep natural language understanding. In *Proceedings of BioNLP 2011 Workshop* (pp. 146–154). Association for Computational Linguistics.

Jurafsky, D., & Martin, J. H. (2014). *Speech and Language Processing*. Pearson London.

Kajbjer, K., Nordberg, R., & Klein, G. O. (2010). Electronic health records in Sweden: From administrative management to clinical decision support. In *IFIP Conference on History of Nordic Computing* (pp. 74–82). Berlin: Springer.

Kandula, S., Curtis, D., & Zeng-Treitler, Q. (2010). A semantic and syntactic text simplification tool for health content. In *AMIA Annual Symposium Proceedings* (Vol. 2010, pp. 366–370).

Kanhov, M. (2014). *Generating Descriptions for Concepts of Swedish SNOMED CT by Implementing a Natural Language Generation System*. Master's thesis, Department of Computer and Systems Sciences, Stockholm University.

Kanhov, M., Feng, X., & Dalianis, H. (2012). Natural language generation from SNOMED specifications. In *In the Proceedings of CLEF 2012 Workshop on Cross-Language Evaluation of Methods, Applications, and Resources for eHealth Document Analysis (CLEFeHealth2012), Rome, September 17–18*.

Karimi, S., Metke-Jimenez, A., Kemp, M., & Wang, C. (2015a). Cadec: A corpus of adverse drug event annotations. *Journal of Biomedical Informatics, 55*, 73–81.

Karimi, S., Wang, C., Metke-Jimenez, A., Gaire, R., & Paris, C. (2015b). Text and data mining techniques in adverse drug reaction detection. *ACM Computing Surveys (CSUR), 47*(4), 56.

Kavuluru, R., Rios, A., & Lu, Y. (2015). An empirical evaluation of supervised learning approaches in assigning diagnosis codes to electronic medical records. *Artificial Intelligence in Medicine, 65*(2), 155–166.

Kelly, L., Goeuriot, L., Suominen, H., Névéol, A., Palotti, J., & Zuccon, G. (2016). Overview of the CLEF eHealth evaluation lab 2016. In *International Conference of the Cross-Language Evaluation Forum for European Languages* (pp. 255–266). Berlin: Springer.

Kholghi, M., Sitbon, L., Zuccon, G., & Nguyen, A. (2015). Active learning: A step towards automating medical concept extraction. *Journal of the American Medical Informatics Association, 23*(2), 289–296.

Koeling, R., Carroll, J., Tate, A. R., & Nicholson, A. (2011). Annotating a corpus of clinical text records for learning to recognize symptoms automatically. In *Proceedings of the 3rd Louhi Workshop on Text and Data Mining of Health Documents* (pp. 43–50).

Kohavi, R. (1995). A study of cross-validation and bootstrap for accuracy estimation and model selection. In *International Joint Conference on Artificial Intelligence (IJCAI)* (pp. 1137–1145).

Kokkinakis, D., Fors, K. L., Björkner, E., & Nordlund, A. (2017). Data collection from persons with mild forms of cognitive impairment and healthy controls-infrastructure for classification and prediction of dementia. In *Proceedings of the 21st Nordic Conference on Computational Linguistics, NoDaLiDa, 22–24 May 2017, Gothenburg, Sweden* (pp. 172–182). Linköping University Electronic Press.

Kokkinakis, D., & Thurin, A. (2007). Anonymisation of Swedish clinical data. In *Conference on Artificial Intelligence in Medicine in Europe* (pp. 237–241). Berlin: Springer.

Koopman, B., Karimi, S., Nguyen, A., McGuire, R., Muscatello, D., Kemp, M., et al. (2015a). Automatic classification of diseases from free-text death certificates for real-time surveillance. *BMC Medical Informatics and Decision Making, 15*(1), 53.

Koopman, B., Zuccon, G., Wagholikar, A., Chu, K., O'Dwyer, J., Nguyen, A., et al. (2015b). Automated reconciliation of radiology reports and discharge summaries. In *AMIA Annual Symposium Proceedings* (Vol. 2015, pp. 775–784). American Medical Informatics Association.

Korkontzelos, I., Mu, T., & Ananiadou, S. (2012). ASCOT: A text mining-based web-service for efficient search and assisted creation of clinical trials. *BMC Medical Informatics and Decision Making, 12*(1), S3.

Kukich, K. (1992). Techniques for automatically correcting words in text. *ACM Computing Surveys (CSUR), 24*(4), 377–439.

Kvist, M., & Velupillai, S. (2014). SCAN: A Swedish clinical abbreviation normalizer. Further development and adaptation to radiology. In *International Conference of the Cross-Language Evaluation Forum for European Languages* (pp. 62–73). Berlin: Springer.

Lafferty, J., McCallum, A., & Pereira, F. (2001). Conditional random fields: Probabilistic models for segmenting and labeling sequence data. In *Proceedings 18th International Conference on Machine Learning* (pp. 282–289). Los Altos, CA: Morgan Kaufmann.

Lagos, K. (2016). *Building an Artifact to Detect Adverse Drug Events in Stockholm EPR Corpus by Using the Stausberg and Hasford's Framework*. Master's thesis, Department of Computer and Systems Sciences, Stockholm University.

Läkemedelsverket. (2012). *Läkemedelsboken 2011–2012, (In Swedish)*. Läkemedelsverket. https://lakemedelsboken.se/pdf/. Accessed 11 Jan 2018.

Lavergne, T., Névéol, A., Robert, A., Grouin, C., Rey, G., & Zweigenbaum, P. (2016). A dataset for ICD-10 coding of death certificates: Creation and usage. *In the Proceedings of the Fifth Workshop on Building and Evaluating Resources for Biomedical Text Mining (BioTxtM 2016), Held in Conjunction with Coling 2016* (pp. 60–69).

Lee, D., Cornet, R., Lau, F., & De Keizer, N. (2013). A survey of SNOMED CT implementations. *Journal of Biomedical Informatics, 46*(1), 87–96.

Lee, D., de Keizer, N., Lau, F., & Cornet, R. (2014). Literature review of SNOMED CT use. *Journal of the American Medical Informatics Association, 21*(e1), e11–e19.

Leonard Westgate, C., Shiner, B., Thompson, P., & Watts, B. V. (2015). Evaluation of veterans' suicide risk with the use of linguistic detection methods. *Psychiatric Services, 66*(10), 1051–1056.

Levenshtein, V. I. (1966). Binary codes capable of correcting deletions, insertions, and reversals. *Soviet Physics Doklady, 10*(8), 707–710.

Lewis, J. D., Schinnar, R., Bilker, W. B., Wang, X., & Strom, B. L. (2007). Validation studies of the health improvement network (THIN) database for pharmacoepidemiology research. *Pharmacoepidemiology and Drug safety, 16*(4), 393–401.

Lingren, T., Deleger, L., Molnar, K., Zhai, H., Meinzen-Derr, J., Kaiser, M., et al. (2014). Evaluating the impact of pre-annotation on annotation speed and potential bias: Natural language processing gold standard development for clinical named entity recognition in clinical trial announcements. *Journal of the American Medical Informatics Association, 21*(3), 406–413.

Liu, H., Aronson, A. R., & Friedman, C. (2002). A study of abbreviations in medline abstracts. In *AMIA Annual Symposium Proceedings* (p. 464). American Medical Informatics Association.

Liu, H., Lussier, Y. A., & Friedman, C. (2001). A study of abbreviations in the UMLS. In *AMIA Annual Symposium Proceedings* (p. 393). American Medical Informatics Association.

Liu, S. (2009). Experiences with and reflections on text summarization tools. *International Journal of Computational Intelligence Systems, 2*(3), 202–218.

Lövestam, E., Velupillai, S., & Kvist, M. (2014). Abbreviations in Swedish clinical text - Use by three professions. *Studies in Health Technology and Informatics, 205*, 720–724. https://doi.org/10.3233/978-1-61499-432-9-720.

Luhn, H. P. (1958). The automatic creation of literature abstracts. *IBM Journal of Research and Development, 2*(2), 159–165.

Luo, Y., Thompson, W. K., Herr, T. M., Zeng, Z., Berendsen, M. A., Jonnalagadda, S. R., et al. (2017). Natural language processing for EHR-based pharmacovigilance: A structured review. *Drug Safety, 40*(11), 1075–1089.

Luo, Y., Uzuner, Ö., & Szolovits, P. (2016). Bridging semantics and syntax with graph algorithms–state-of-the-art of extracting biomedical relations. *Briefings in Bioinformatics, 18*(1), 160–178.

Mani, I., & Maybury, M. T. (1999). *Advances in Automatic Text Summarization* (Vol. 293). Cambridge, MA: MIT Press.

Manning, C. D., Raghavan, P., & Schutze, H. (2008). *Introduction to Information Retrieval.* Cambridge: Cambridge University Press.

Marciniak, M., & Mykowiecka, A. (2014). Terminology extraction from medical texts in Polish. *Journal of Biomedical Semantics, 5*(1), 24.

Martinez, D., & Li, Y. (2011). Information extraction from pathology reports in a hospital setting. In *Proceedings of the 20th ACM International Conference on Information and Knowledge Management* (pp. 1877–1882). New York: ACM.

McMorrow, L. (1998). Breaking the Greco-Roman mold in medical writing: The many languages of 20th century medicine. In *Translation and Medicine* 13–27, John Benjamins Publishing Company/Amsterdam Philadelphia.

Mellner, C., Selander, H., & Wolodarski, J. (1974). The Karolinska hospital information system. *Methods of Information in Medicine, 13*(3), 125–140.

Metzger, M.-H., Durand, T., Lallich, S., Salamon, R., & Castets, P. (2012). The use of regional platforms for managing electronic health records for the production of regional public health indicators in France. *BMC Medical Informatics and Decision Making, 12*(1), 28.

Metzger, M.-H., Tvardik, N., Gicquel, Q., Bouvry, C., Poulet, E., & Potinet-Pagliaroli, V. (2016). Use of emergency department electronic medical records for automated epidemiological surveillance of suicide attempts: a French pilot study. *International Journal of Methods in Psychiatric Research, 26*(2), 1–10.

Meystre, S., Friedlin, J., South, B., Shen, S., & Samore, M. (2010). Automatic de-identification of textual documents in the electronic health record: A review of recent research. *BMC Medical Research Methodology, 10*(1), 70.

Meystre, S. M. (2015). De-identification of unstructured clinical data for patient privacy protection. In *Medical Data Privacy Handbook* (pp. 697–716). Berlin: Springer.

Meystre, S. M., Lovis, C., Bürkle, T., Tognola, G., Budrionis, A., & Lehmann, C. U. (2017). Clinical data reuse or secondary use: Current status and potential future progress. *Yearbook of Medical Informatics, 26*(01), 38–52.

Meystre, S. M., Savova, G. K., Kipper-Schuler, K. C., & Hurdle, J. F. (2008). Extracting information from textual documents in the electronic health record: A review of recent research. *Yearbook of Medical Informatics, 35*, 128–144.

Meystre, S. M., Shen, S., Hofmann, D., & Gundlapalli, A. V. (2014). Can physicians recognize their own patients in de-identified notes? In *MIE-Medical Informatics Europe* (pp. 778–782).

Mikolov, T., Sutskever, I., Chen, K., Corrado, G. S., & Dean, J. (2013). Distributed representations of words and phrases and their compositionality. In *Advances in Neural Information Processing Systems* (pp. 3111–3119).

Miller, A. C. (2006). Jundi-Shapur, bimaristans, and the rise of academic medical centres. *Journal of the Royal Society of Medicine, 99*(12), 615–617.

Mitkov, R. (2014). *Anaphora Resolution: The State of the Art*. Routledge.

Mitkov, R. (2005). *The Oxford Handbook of Computational Linguistics*. Oxford: Oxford University Press.

Moen, H. (2016). *Distributional Semantic Models for Clinical Text Applied to Health Record Summarization*. PhD thesis, Department of Computer and Information Science, Norwegian University of Science and Technology, NTNU.

Moen, H., Peltonen, L.-M., Heimonen, J., Airola, A., Pahikkala, T., Salakoski, T., et al. (2016). Comparison of automatic summarisation methods for clinical free text notes. *Artificial Intelligence in Medicine, 67*, 25–37.

Morante, R., & Daelemans, W. (2009). A metalearning approach to processing the scope of negation. In *CoNLL '09: Proceedings of the Thirteenth Conference on Computational Natural Language Learning* (pp. 21–29). Association for Computational Linguistics. ISBN 978-1-932432-29-9.

Moriyama, I. M., Loy, R. M., Robb-Smith, A. H., Rosenberg, H. M., & Hoyert, D. L. (2011). *History of the Statistical Classification of Diseases and Causes of Death*. US Department of Health and Human Services, Centers for Disease Control and Prevention, National Center for Health Statistics.

Mowery, D. L., South, B. R., Christensen, L., Leng, J., Peltonen, L.-M., Salanterä, S., et al. (2016). Normalizing acronyms and abbreviations to aid patient understanding of clinical texts: ShARe/CLEF eHealth Challenge 2013, Task 2. *Journal of Biomedical Semantics, 7*(1), 43.

Mutalik, P. G., Deshpande, A., & Nadkarni, P. M. (2001). Use of general-purpose negation detection to augment concept indexing of medical documents. *Journal of the American Medical Informatics Association, 8*(6), 598–609.

Napolitano, G., Marshall, A., Hamilton, P., & Gavin, A. T. (2016). Machine learning classification of surgical pathology reports and chunk recognition for information extraction noise reduction. *Artificial Intelligence in Medicine, 70*, 77–83.

Neamatullah, I., Douglass, M. M., Li-wei, H. L., Reisner, A., Villarroel, M., Long, W. J., et al. (2008). Automated de-identification of free-text medical records. *BMC Medical Informatics and Decision Making, 8*(1), 1.

Nebeker, J. R., Barach, P., & Samore, M. H. (2004). Clarifying adverse drug events: A clinician's guide to terminology, documentation, and reporting. *Annals of Internal Medicine, 140*(10), 795–801.

Névéol, A., Dalianis, H., Savova, G., & Zweigenbaum, P. (2018). Clinical natural language processing in languages other than english: opportunities and challenges. *Journal of Biomedical Semantics, 9*(12), 1–13.

Neves, M., & Leser, U. (2012). A survey on annotation tools for the biomedical literature. *Briefings in Bioinformatics, 15*(2), 327–340.

Nguyen, A., Lawley, M., Hansen, D., & Colquist, S. (2011). Structured pathology reporting for cancer from free text: Lung cancer case study. *Electronic Journal of Health Informatics, 7*(1), 8.

Nguyen, A. N., Lawley, M. J., Hansen, D. P., Bowman, R. V., Clarke, B. E., Duhig, E. E., et al. (2010). Symbolic rule-based classification of lung cancer stages from free-text pathology reports. *Journal of the American Medical Informatics Association, 17*(4), 440–445.

Nguyen, A. N., Moore, J., O'Dwyer, J., & Philpot, S. (2015). Assessing the utility of automatic cancer registry notifications data extraction from free-text pathology reports. In *AMIA Annual Symposium Proceedings* (Vol. 2015, p. 953). American Medical Informatics Association.

Nguyen, A. N., Moore, J., O'Dwyer, J., & Philpot, S. (2016). Automated cancer registry notifications: validation of a medical text analytics system for identifying patients with cancer from a state-wide pathology repository. In *AMIA Annual Symposium Proceedings* (pp. 964–973). American Medical Informatics Association.

Nilsson, I. (2007). *Medicinsk dokumentation genom tiderna: En studie av den svenska patientjournalens utveckling under 1700-talet, 1800-talet och 1900-talet*. Doctoral thesis, Doktorsavhandling, Enheten för medicinens historia, Medicinska fakulteten, Lunds universitet, In Swedish.

Nilsson, I., & Nilsson, P. (2003). Medicinsk dokumentation genom tiderna. *Läkartidningen, 100*(51–52), 6–4304.

Nivre, J., de Marneffe, M.-C., Ginter, F., Goldberg, Y., Hajič, J., Manning, C. D., et al. (2016). Universal dependencies v1: A multilingual treebank collection. In *Proceedings of the Tenth International Conference on Language Resources and Evaluation, LREC 2016* (pp. 1659–1666). http://www.lrec-conf.org/proceedings/lrec2016/pdf/348_Paper.pdf [www.lrec-conf.org].

Nivre, J., Hall, J., & Nilsson, J. (2006). MaltParser: A data-driven parser-generator for dependency parsing. In *Proceedings of the Fifth International Conference on Language Resources and Evaluation, LREC 2006* (pp. 2216–2219). http://www.lrec-conf.org/proceedings/lrec2006/pdf/162_pdf.pdf. Accessed 11 Jan 2018.

Nizamuddin, N., & Dalianis, H. (2014). Detection of spelling errors in Swedish clinical text. In *1st Nordic Workshop on Evaluation of Spellchecking and Proofing Tools (NorWEST2014), SLTC 2014*.

North, M. (2002). The Hippocratic Oath, National Library of Medicine. *History of Medicine Division, United States National Library of Medicine, National Institutes of Health*. http://www.nlm.nih.gov/hmd/greek/greek_oath.html.

Nygren, E., & Henriksson, P. (1992). Reading the medical record. I. Analysis of physician's ways of reading the medical record. *Computer Methods and Programs in Biomedicine, 39*(1), 1–12.

Nygren, E., Johnson, M., & Henriksson, P. (1992). Reading the medical record. II. Design of a human-computer interface for basic reading of computerized medical records. *Computer Methods and Programs in Biomedicine, 39*, 13–25.

Nygren, E., Wyatt, J. C., & Wright, P. (1998). Helping clinicians to find data and avoid delays. *The Lancet, 352*(9138), 1462–1466.

Olsson, F. (2008). *Bootstrapping Named Entity Annotation by Means of Active Machine Learning: A Method for Creating Corpora*. PhD thesis, Department of Swedish Language, University of Gothenburg.

Olsson, F. (2009). *A Literature Survey of Active Machine Learning in the Context of Natural Language Processing*. Technical report, Swedish Institute of Computer Science.

Olsson, M. (2011). *Vem begriper patientjournalen? (In Swedish)*. Bachelor's thesis, Linnaeus University.

Ou, Y., & Patrick, J. (2014). Automatic population of structured reports from narrative pathology reports. In *Proceedings of the Seventh Australasian Workshop on Health Informatics and Knowledge Management* (Vol. 153, pp. 41–50). Australian Computer Society, Inc.

Pakhomov, S., Pedersen, T., & Chute, C. G. (2005). Abbreviation and acronym disambiguation in clinical discourse. In *AMIA Annual Symposium Proceedings* (Vol. 2005, p. 589). American Medical Informatics Association.

Pantazos, K., Lauesen, S., & Lippert, S. (2016). Preserving medical correctness, readability and consistency in de-identified health records. *Health Informatics Journal, 23*(4), 291–303.

Patrick, J., & Li, M. (2010). High accuracy information extraction of medication information from clinical notes: 2009 i2b2 medication extraction challenge. *Journal of the American Medical Informatics Association, 17*(5), 524–527.

Patrick, J., & Nguyen, D. (2011). Automated proof reading of clinical notes. In *PACLIC, 25th Pacific Asia Conference on Language, Information and Computation* (pp. 303–312).

Perera, G., Broadbent, M., Callard, F., Chang, C.-K., Downs, J., Dutta, R., et al. (2016). Cohort profile of the South London and Maudsley NHS Foundation Trust Biomedical Research Centre (SLaM BRC) Case Register: current status and recent enhancement of an electronic mental health record-derived data resource. *BMJ Open, 6*(3), e008721.

Pérez, A., Weegar, R., Casillas, A., Gojenola, K., Oronoz, M., & Dalianis, H. (2017). Semi-supervised medical entity recognition: A study on Spanish and Swedish clinical corpora. *Journal of Biomedical Informatics, 71*, 16–30.

Perotte, A., Pivovarov, R., Natarajan, K., Weiskopf, N., Wood, F., & Elhadad, N. (2014). Diagnosis code assignment: Models and evaluation metrics. *Journal of the American Medical Informatics Association, 21*(2), 231–237.

Pestian, J. P., Brew, C., Matykiewicz, P., Hovermale, D. J., Johnson, N., Cohen, K. B., et al. (2007). A shared task involving multi-label classification of clinical free text. In *Proceedings of the Workshop on BioNLP 2007: Biological, Translational, and Clinical Language Processing* (pp. 97–104). Association for Computational Linguistics.

Pirinen, T., & Lindén, K. (2010). Creating and weighting hunspell dictionaries as finite-state automata. *Investigationes Linguisticae, 21*, 1–16.

Pivovarov, R., & Elhadad, N. (2015). Automated methods for the summarization of electronic health records. *Journal of the American Medical Informatics Association, 22*(5), 938–947.

Plaisant, C., Mushlin, R., Snyder, A., Li, J., Heller, D., & Shneiderman, B. (1998). Lifelines: Using visualization to enhance navigation and analysis of patient records. In *AMIA Annual Symposium Proceedings* (pp. 76–80). American Medical Informatics Association.

Portet, F., Reiter, E., Gatt, A., Hunter, J., Sripada, S., Freer, Y., et al. (2009). Automatic generation of textual summaries from neonatal intensive care data. *Artificial Intelligence, 173*(7–8), 789–816.

Pradhan, S., Elhadad, N., Chapman, W. W., Manandhar, S., & Savova, G. (2014). Semeval-2014 task 7: Analysis of clinical text. In *SemEval@ COLING* (pp. 54–62).

Pratt, A. W., & Pacak, M. G. (1969). Automated processing of medical English. In *Proceedings of the 1969 Conference on Computational Linguistics* (pp. 1–23). Association for Computational Linguistics.

Proux, D., Hagège, C., Gicquel, Q., Pereira, S., Darmoni, S., Segond, F., et al. (2011). Architecture and systems for monitoring hospital acquired infections inside a hospital information workflow. In *Proceedings of the Workshop on Biomedical Natural Language Processing. USA: Portland, Oregon* (p. 43e48). Citeseer.

Pustejovsky, J., Castano, J. M., Ingria, R., Sauri, R., Gaizauskas, R. J., Setzer, A., et al. (2003). TimeML: Robust specification of event and temporal expressions in text. *New Directions in Question Answering, 3*, 28–34.

Pustejovsky, J., & Stubbs, A. (2012). *Natural Language Annotation for Machine Learning*. O'Reilly Media, Inc. Beijing.

Ramesh, B. P., Houston, T. K., Brandt, C., Fang, H., & Yu, H. (2013). Improving patients' electronic health record comprehension with NoteAid. In *Medinfo* (pp. 714–718).

Roberts, A., Gaizauskas, R., Hepple, M., Demetriou, G., Guo, Y., Roberts, I., et al. (2009). Building a semantically annotated corpus of clinical texts. *Journal of Biomedical Informatics, 42*(5), 950–966.

Roberts, A., Gaizauskas, R., Hepple, M., & Guo, Y. (2008). Mining clinical relationships from patient narratives. *BMC Bioinformatics, 9*(11), 1.

Roberts, K., Simpson, M., Demner-Fushman, D., Voorhees, E., & Hersh, W. (2016). State-of-the-art in biomedical literature retrieval for clinical cases: A survey of the TREC 2014 CDS track. *Information Retrieval Journal, 19*(1–2), 113–148.

Rokach, L., Romano, R., & Maimo, O. (2008). Negation recognition in medical narrative reports. *Information Retrieval Journal, 11*(6), 499–538.

Roller, R., & Stevenson, M. (2014). Self-supervised relation extraction using UMLS. In *International Conference of the Cross-Language Evaluation Forum for European Languages* (pp. 116–127). Berlin: Springer.

Roller, R., Uszkoreit, H., Xu, F., Seiffe, L., Mikhailov, M., Staeck, O., et al. (2016). A fine-grained corpus annotation schema of German nephrology records. In *Proceedings of the Clinical Natural Language Processing Workshop, Osaka, Japan, December 11–17* (pp. 69–77).

Roque, F. S., Jensen, P. B., Schmock, H., Dalgaard, M., Andreatta, M., Hansen, T., et al. (2011a). Using electronic patient records to discover disease correlations and stratify patient cohorts. *PLOS Computational Biology, 7*(8), e1002141.

Roque, F. S., Jensen, P. B., Schmock, H., Dalgaard, M., Andreatta, M., Hansen, T., et al. (2011b). Using electronic patient records to discover disease correlations and stratify patient cohorts. *PLOS Computational Biology, 7*(8), e1002141.

Roque, F. S., Slaughter, L., & Tkatšenko, A. (2010). A comparison of several key information visualization systems for secondary use of electronic health record content. In *Proceedings of the NAACL HLT 2010 Second Louhi Workshop on Text and Data Mining of Health Documents* (pp. 76–83). Association for Computational Linguistics.

Rosell, M. (2009). *Text Clustering Exploration: Swedish Text Representation and Clustering Results Unraveled*. PhD thesis, Computer Science and Communications, CSC, KTH.

Ruch, P., Robert, B., & Antoine, G. (2003). Using lexical disambiguation and named-entity recognition to improve spelling correction in the electronic patient record. *Artificial Intelligence in Medicine, 29*(1), 169–184.

Saeed, M., Villarroel, M., Reisner, A. T., Clifford, G., Lehman, L.-W., Moody, G., et al. (2011). Multiparameter intelligent monitoring in intensive care II (MIMIC-II): A public-access intensive care unit database. *Critical Care Medicine, 39*(5), 952.

Sahlgren, M. (2006). *The Word-Space Model: Using Distributional Analysis to Represent Syntagmatic and Paradigmatic Relations Between Words in High-Dimensional Vector Spaces*. PhD thesis, Department of Linguistics, Stockholm University.

SALAR. (2014). Swedish Association of Local Authorities and Regions: Vårdrelaterade infektioner framgångsfaktorer som förebygger. Stockholm, Sweden. http://webbutik.skl.se/bilder/artiklar/pdf/978-91-7585-109-9.pdf. Accessed 10 Apr 2014. ISBN 978-91-7585-109-9.

Santiso, S., Pérez, A., Gojenola, K., Taldea, I. X. A., Casillas, A., & Oronoz, M. (2014). Adverse drug event prediction combining shallow analysis and machine learning. In *Proceedings of the 5th International Workshop on Health Text Mining and Information Analysis (Louhi)@ EACL* (pp. 85–89).

Sarker, A., Mollá, D., & Paris, C. (2013). An approach for query-focused text summarisation for evidence based medicine. In *Artificial Intelligence in Medicine* (pp. 295–304). Berlin: Springer.

Saurí, R., & Pustejovsky, J. (2009). Factbank: A corpus annotated with event factuality. *Language Resources and Evaluation, 43*(3), 227–268.

Savova, G. K., Masanz, J. J., Ogren, P. V., Zheng, J., Sohn, S., Kipper-Schuler, K. C., et al. (2010). Mayo clinical text analysis and knowledge extraction system (cTAKES): Architecture, component evaluation and applications. *Journal of the American Medical Informatics Association, 17*(5), 507–513.

Scharber, W. (2007). Evaluation of open source text mining tools for cancer surveillance. *CDC, 24*, 28. https://www.cdc.gov/cancer/npcr/pdf/aerro/text_mining_tools.pdf. Accessed 11 Jan 2018.

Settles, B. (2009). *Active Learning Literature Survey.* Computer Sciences Technical report 1648, University of Wisconsin–Madison.

Siklósi, B., Novák, A., & Prószéky, G. (2014). Resolving abbreviations in clinical texts without pre-existing structured resources. In *Fourth Workshop on Building and Evaluating Resources for Health and Biomedical Text Processing, LREC* (Vol. 2014).

Siklósi, B., Novák, A., & Prószéky, G. (2016). Context-aware correction of spelling errors in Hungarian medical documents. *Computer Speech & Language, 35*, 219–233.
Singh, H., Knudsen Sollie, M., Orholm Solhøi, E., & Sverre Syberg, F. (2015). *Information Extraction: The Case of Kreftregisteret, (In Norwegian)*. Bachelor's thesis, Westerdals Oslo ACT.
Skeppstedt, M. (2011). Negation detection in Swedish clinical text: An adaption of NegEx to Swedish. *Journal of Biomedical Semantics, 2*(Suppl 3), S3.
Skeppstedt, M. (2013). Annotating named entities in clinical text by combining pre-annotation and active learning. In *ACL (Student Research Workshop)* (pp. 74–80).
Skeppstedt, M. (2015). *Extracting Clinical Findings from Swedish Health Record Text*. PhD thesis, Department of Computer and Systems Sciences, Stockholm University.
Skeppstedt, M., Kvist, M., & Dalianis, H. (2012). Rule-based entity recognition and coverage of SNOMED CT in Swedish clinical text. In *Proceedings of the Eighth International Conference on Language Resources and Evaluation, LREC 2012* (pp. 1250–1257).
Skeppstedt, M., Kvist, M., Nilsson, G., & Dalianis, H. (2014). Automatic recognition of disorders, findings, pharmaceuticals and body structures from clinical text: An annotation and machine learning study. In *Journal of Biomedical Informatics, 49*, 148–158.
Skeppstedt, M., Paradis, C., & Kerren, A. (2017). PAL, a tool for pre-annotation and active learning. *Journal for Language Technology and Computational Linguistics, 31*(1), 91–110.
Smith, K., Megyesi, B., Velupillai, S., & Kvist, M. (2014). Professional language in Swedish clinical text: Linguistic characterization and comparative studies. *Nordic Journal of Linguistics, 37*(02), 297–323.
Socialstyrelsen. (2010). The National Board of Health and Welfare, Kodningskvalitet i patientregistret, Slutenvård 2008, (In Swedish). http://www.socialstyrelsen.se/Lists/Artikelkatalog/Attachments/18082/2010-6-27.pdf.
South, B. R., Shen, S., Jones, M., Garvin, J., Samore, M. H., Chapman, W. W., et al. (2009). Developing a manually annotated clinical document corpus to identify phenotypic information for inflammatory bowel disease. *BMC Bioinformatics, 10*(9), S12.
Spasić, I., Livsey, J., Keane, J. A., & Nenadić, G. (2014). Text mining of cancer-related information: Review of current status and future directions. *International Journal of Medical Informatics, 83*(9), 605–623. http://dx.doi.org/10.1016/j.ijmedinf.2014.06.009. Accessed 11 Jan 2018.
Spat, S., Cadonna, B., Rakovac, I., Gütl, C., Leitner, H., Stark, G., et al. (2008). Enhanced information retrieval from narrative German-language clinical text documents using automated document classification. *Studies in Health Technology and Informatics, 136*, 473.
Spyns, P. (1996). Natural language processing in medicine: An overview. *Methods of Information in Medicine, 35*(4–5), 285–301.
Stanfill, M. H., Williams, M., Fenton, S. H., Jenders, R. A., & Hersh, W. R. (2010). A systematic literature review of automated clinical coding and classification systems. *Journal of the American Medical Informatics Association, 17*(6), 646–651.
Stausberg, J., & Hasford, J. (2011). Drug-related admissions and hospital-acquired adverse drug events in Germany: A longitudinal analysis from 2003 to 2007 of ICD-10-coded routine data. *BMC Health Research, 11*(1), 1.
Stenetorp, P., Pyysalo, S., Topić, G., Ohta, T., Ananiadou, S., & Tsujii, J. (2012). BRAT: A web-based tool for NLP-assisted text annotation. In *Proceedings of the Demonstrations at the 13th Conference of the European Chapter of the Association for Computational Linguistics* (pp. 102–107). Association for Computational Linguistics.
Strötgen, J., & Gertz, M. (2010). HeidelTime: High quality rule-based extraction and normalization of temporal expressions. In *Proceedings of the 5th International Workshop on Semantic Evaluation* (pp. 321–324). Association for Computational Linguistics.
Stumpf, S., Rajaram, V., Li, L., Wong, W.-K., Burnett, M., Dietterich, T., et al. (2009). Interacting meaningfully with machine learning systems: Three experiments. *International Journal of Human-Computer Studies, 67*(8), 639–662.

Styler IV, W., Bethard, S., Finan, S., Palmer, M., Pradhan, S., de Groen, P., et al. (2014). Temporal annotation in the clinical domain. *Transactions of the Association for Computational Linguistics, 2*, 143–154. https://tacl2013.cs.columbia.edu/ojs/index.php/tacl/article/view/305. Accessed 11 Jan 2018. ISSN 2307-387X.

Sun, W., Rumshisky, A., & Uzuner, Ö. (2013a). Evaluating temporal relations in clinical text: 2012 i2b2 challenge. *Journal of the American Medical Informatics Association, 20*(5), 806–813.

Sun, W., Rumshisky, A., & Uzuner, Ö. (2013b). Temporal reasoning over clinical text: The state of the art. *Journal of the American Medical Informatics Association, 20*(5), 814–819.

Suominen, H. (2012). Towards an international electronic repository and virtual laboratory of open data and open-source software for telehealth research: Comparison of international, Australian and Finnish privacy policies. *Studies in Health Technology and Informatics, 182*, 153–160.

Suominen, H., Ginter, F., Pyysalo, S., Airola, A., Pahikkala, T., Salanterä, S., et al. (2008). Machine learning to automate the assignment of diagnosis codes to free-text radiology reports: A method description. In *Proceedings of the ICML/UAI/COLT Workshop on Machine Learning for Health-Care Applications*.

Suominen, H., Müller, H., Ohno-Machado, L., Salanterä, S., Schreier, G., & Hanlen, L. (2017). Prerequisites for International Exchanges of Health Information: Comparison of Australian, Austrian, Finnish, Swiss, and US Privacy Policies. Studies in Health Technology and Informatics, Vol 245, pp. 1312.

Suominen, H., Salanterä, S., Velupillai, S., Chapman, W. W., Savova, G., Elhadad, N., et al. (2013). Overview of the ShARe/CLEF eHealth Evaluation Lab 2013. In *Information Access Evaluation. Multilinguality, Multimodality, and Visualization* (pp. 212–231). Berlin: Springer.

Sweeney, L. (1996). Replacing personally-identifying information in medical records, the scrub system. In *Proceedings of the AMIA Annual Fall Symposium* (p. 333). American Medical Informatics Association.

Sweeney, L. (2002). k-anonymity: A model for protecting privacy. *International Journal of Uncertainty, Fuzziness and Knowledge-Based Systems, 10*(05), 557–570.

Syed, I. B. (2002). Islamic medicine: 1000 years ahead of its times. *Journal of the International Society of the History of Islamic Medicine, 2*, 2–9.

Szarvas, G. (2008). Hedge classification in biomedical texts with a weakly supervised selection of keywords. In *Proceedings of ACL-08: HLT*, Columbus, Ohio, June 2008 (pp. 281–289). Association for Computational Linguistics. http://www.aclweb.org/anthology/P/P08/P08-1033.

Tang, R., Ouyang, L., Li, C., He, Y., Griffin, M., Taghian, A., et al. (2018). Machine learning to parse breast pathology reports in Chinese. *Breast Cancer Research and Treatment*, 1–8, https://doi.org/10.1007/s10549-018-4668-3.

Tanushi, H., Dalianis, H., & Nilsson, G. (2011). Calculating prevalence of comorbidity and comorbidity combinations with diabetes in hospital care in Sweden using a health care record database. In *Proceedings of the LOUHI 2011, Third International Workshop on Health Document Text Mining and Information Analysis, Co-located with AIME 2011 Bled, Slovenia, July 6, 2011, CEUR-WS* (Vol. 744, pp. 59–66). ISSN 1613-0073

Tanushi, H., Kvist, M., & Sparrelid, E. (2014). Detection of healthcare-associated urinary tract infection in Swedish electronic health records. *Studies in Health Technology and Informatics, 207*, 330–339.

Temkin, O. (1962). Byzantine medicine: Tradition and empiricism. *Dumbarton Oaks Papers, 16*, 95–115.

Tengstrand, L., Megyesi, B., Henriksson, A., Duneld, M., & Kvist, M. (2014). EACL – Expansion of abbreviations in clinical text. In *Proceedings of the 3rd Workshop on Predicting and Improving Text Readability for Target Reader Populations (PITR)* (pp. 94–103). Association for Computational Linguistics.

Tissot, H. C. (2016). *Normalisation of Imprecise Temporal Expressions Extracted from Text*. PhD thesis, Computer Science at the Federal University of Paraná.

Torgersson, O., & Falkman, G. (2002). Using text generation to access clinical data in a variety of contexts. *Studies in Health Technology and Informatics*, Vol 90, 460–465.

Tran, T., Luo, W., Phung, D., Harvey, R., Berk, M., Kennedy, R. L., et al. (2014). Risk stratification using data from electronic medical records better predicts suicide risks than clinician assessments. *BMC Psychiatry, 14*(1), 76.

Uzuner, Ö., Bodnari, A., Shen, S., Forbush, T., Pestian, J., & South, B. R. (2012). Evaluating the state of the art in coreference resolution for electronic medical records. *Journal of the American Medical Informatics Association, 19*(5), 786–791.

Uzuner, Ö., Luo, Y., & Szolovits, P. (2007). Evaluating the state-of-the-art in automatic de-identification. *Journal of the American Medical Informatics Association, 14*(5), 550–563.

Uzuner, Ö., Sibanda, T. C., Luo, Y., & Szolovits, P. (2008). A de-identifier for medical discharge summaries. *Artificial Intelligence in Medicine, 42*(1), 13–35.

Uzuner, Ö., Solti, I., & Cadag, E. (2010). Extracting medication information from clinical text. *Journal of the American Medical Informatics Association, 17*(5), 514–518.

Uzuner, Ö., South, B. R., Shen, S., & DuVall, S. L. (2011). 2010 i2b2/va challenge on concepts, assertions, and relations in clinical text. *Journal of the American Medical Informatics Association, 18*(5), 552–556.

Van Rijsbergen, C. J. (1979). *Information Retrieval*. Butterworth & Co. http://www.dcs.glasgow.ac.uk/Keith/Preface.html. Accessed 11 Jan 2018.

Van Vleck, T. T., & Elhadad, N. (2010). Corpus-based problem selection for EHR note summarization. In *AMIA Annual Symposium Proceedings* (Vol. 2010, p. 817). American Medical Informatics Association.

Velupillai, S. (2011). Automatic classification of factuality levels: A case study on Swedish diagnoses and the impact of local context. In *Fourth International Symposium on Languages in Biology and Medicine, LBM 2011*.

Velupillai, S. (2012). *Shades of Certainty: Annotation and Classification of Swedish Medical Records*. PhD thesis, Stockholm University.

Velupillai, S. (2014). Temporal expressions in Swedish medical text – A pilot study. In *Proceedings of BioNLP 2014*, Baltimore, MD, June 2014 (pp. 88–92). Association for Computational Linguistics. http://www.aclweb.org/anthology/W14-3413. Accessed 11 Jan 2018.

Velupillai, S., Dalianis, H., Hassel, M., & Nilsson, G. H. (2009). Developing a standard for de-identifying electronic patient records written in Swedish: Precision, recall and F-measure in a manual and computerized annotation trial. *International Journal of Medical Informatics, 78*(12), e19–e26.

Velupillai, S., Dalianis, H., & Kvist, M. (2011). Factuality levels of diagnoses in Swedish clinical text. In *MIE-Medical Informatics Europe* (pp. 559–563). http://dx.doi.org/10.3233/978-1-60750-806-9-559.

Velupillai, S. & Kvist, M. (2012). Fine-grained certainty level annotations used for coarser-grained e-health scenarios. In *International Conference on Intelligent Text Processing and Computational Linguistics* (pp. 450–461). Berlin: Springer.

Velupillai, S., Mowery, D., South, B. R., Kvist, M., & Dalianis, H. (2015). Recent advances in clinical natural language processing in support of semantic analysis. *Yearbook of Medical Informatics, 10*(1), 183.

Velupillai, S., Skeppstedt, M., Kvist, M., Mowery, D., Chapman, B. E., Dalianis, H., et al. (2014). Cue-based assertion classification for Swedish clinical text–Developing a lexicon for pyConTextSwe. *Artificial Intelligence in Medicine, 61*(3), 137–144.

Vincze, V., Szarvas, G., Farkas, R., Móra, G., & Csirik, J. (2008). The BioScope Corpus: Biomedical texts annotated for uncertainty, negation and their scopes. *BMC Bioinformatics, 9*(Suppl 11), S9.

Voorhees, E. M. (2001). The philosophy of information retrieval evaluation. In *Evaluation of Cross-Language Information Retrieval Systems* (pp. 355–370). Berlin: Springer.

Voorhees, E. M., & Hersh, W. R. (2012). Overview of the TREC 2012 medical records track. In *Proceedings of Text REtrieval Conference (TREC)*.

Wang, T. D., Wongsuphasawat, K., Plaisant, C., & Shneiderman, B. (2011). Extracting insights from electronic health records: Case studies, a visual analytics process model, and design recommendations. *Journal of Medical Systems, 35*(5), 1135–1152.

Wang, X., Hripcsak, G., Markatou, M., & Friedman, C. (2009). Active computerized pharmacovigilance using natural language processing, statistics, and electronic health records: A feasibility study. *Journal of the American Medical Informatics Association, 16*(3), 328–337.

Wang, Y., Coiera, E., Runciman, W., & Magrabi, F. (2017). Using multiclass classification to automate the identification of patient safety incident reports by type and severity. *BMC Medical Informatics and Decision Making, 17*(1), 84.

Wang, Y., & Patrick, J. (2009). Cascading classifiers for named entity recognition in clinical notes. In *Proceedings of the Workshop on Biomedical Information Extraction* (pp. 42–49). Association for Computational Linguistics.

Wang, Y., Patrick, J., Miller, G., & O'Hallaran, J. (2008). A computational linguistics motivated mapping of ICPC-2 PLUS to SNOMED CT. *BMC Medical Informatics and Decision Making, 8*(1), S5.

Warrer, P., Hansen, E. H., Juhl-Jensen, L., & Aagaard, L. (2012). Using text-mining techniques in electronic patient records to identify ADRS from medicine use. *British Journal of Clinical Pharmacology, 73*(5), 674–684.

Weed, L. L. (1968). Medical records that guide and teach. *New England Journal of Medicine, 278*(12), 652–657.

Weegar, R., & Dalianis, H. (2015). Creating a rule based system for text mining of Norwegian breast cancer pathology reports. In *Sixth International Workshop in Health Text Mining and Information Analysis (LOUHI), Held in Conjunction with EMNLP 2015, Lisbon, Portugal* (pp. 73–78).

Weegar, R., Kvist, M., Sundström, K., Brunak, S., & Dalianis, H. (2015). Finding cervical cancer symptoms in Swedish clinical text using a machine learning approach and NegEx. In *AMIA Annual Symposium Proceedings* (Vol. 2015, pp. 1296–1305). American Medical Informatics Association.

Weegar, R., Nygård, J., & Dalianis, H. (2017). Efficient encoding of pathology reports using natural language processing. In *Proceedings of Recent Advances in Natural Language Processing, RANLP 2017, Varna, Bulgaria* (pp. 778–783).

Wester, K., Jönsson, A. K., Spigset, O., Druid, H., & Hägg, S. (2008). Incidence of fatal adverse drug reactions: A population based study. *British Journal of Clinical Pharmacology, 65*(4), 573–579.

Winau, R. (1994). The Hippocratic Oath and ethics in medicine. *Forensic Science International, 69*(3), 285–289.

Wong, W., & Glance, D. (2011). Statistical semantic and clinician confidence analysis for real-time clinical progress note cleaning. *Artificial Intelligence in Medicine, 53*, 171–180.

Wong, W., Liu, W., & Bennamoun, M. (2006). Integrated scoring for spelling error correction, abbreviation expansion and case restoration in dirty text. In *Proceedings of the Fifth Australasian conference on Data Mining and Analytics* (Vol. 61, pp. 83–89). Australian Computer Society, Inc.

Wu, Y., Rosenbloom, S. T., Denny, J. C., Miller, R. A., Mani, S., Giuse, D. A., et al. (2011). Detecting abbreviations in discharge summaries using machine learning methods. In *AMIA Annual Symposium Proceedings* (Vol. 2011, p. 1541). American Medical Informatics Association.

Xu, H., Stetson, P. D., & Friedman, C. (2007). A study of abbreviations in clinical notes. In *AMIA Annual Symposium Proceedings* (Vol. 2007, p. 821). American Medical Informatics Association.

Yala, A., Barzilay, R., Salama, L., Griffin, M., Sollender, G., Bardia, A., et al. (2017). Using machine learning to parse breast pathology reports. *Breast Cancer Research and Treatment, 161*(2), 203–211.

Zeng, Q. T., Redd, D., Rindflesch, T. C., & Nebeker, J. R. (2012). Synonym, topic model and predicate-based query expansion for retrieving clinical documents. In *AMIA Annual Symposium Proceedings*.

Zhang, S., Kang, T., Zhang, X., Wen, D., Elhadad, N., & Lei, J. (2016). Speculation detection for Chinese clinical notes: Impacts of word segmentation and embedding models. *Journal of Biomedical Informatics, 60*, 334–341.

Zhao, D., & Weng, C. (2011). Combining PubMed knowledge and EHR data to develop a weighted Bayesian network for pancreatic cancer prediction. *Journal of Biomedical Informatics, 44*, 859–868.

Zhou, L., Friedman, C., Parsons, S., & Hripcsak, G. (2005). System architecture for temporal information extraction, representation and reasoning in clinical narrative reports. In *AMIA Annual Symposium Proceedings* (pp. 869–873).

Zhou, L., & Hripcsak, G. (2007). Temporal reasoning with medical data–A review with emphasis on medical natural language processing. *Journal of Biomedical Informatics, 40*(2), 183–202.

Zubke, M. (2017). Classification based extraction of numeric values from clinical narratives. In *Proceedings of RANLP Workshop on Biomedical Natural Language Processing* (pp. 24–31).

Index

H. Dalianis, *Clinical Text Mining*, https://doi.org/10.1007/978-3-319-78503-5

: United States
ısters